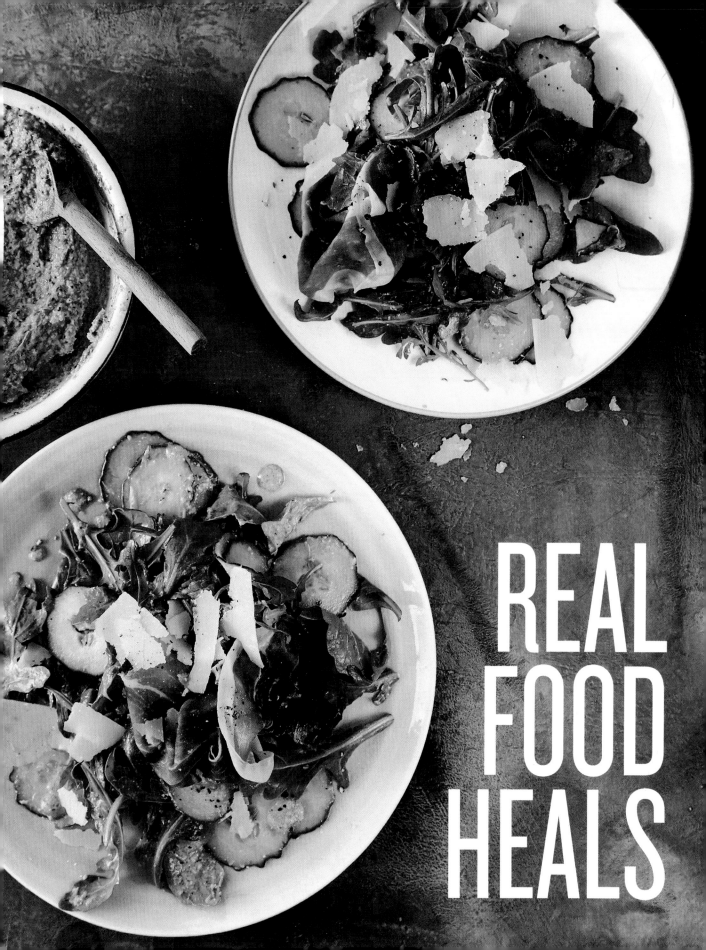

REAL
FOOD
HEALS

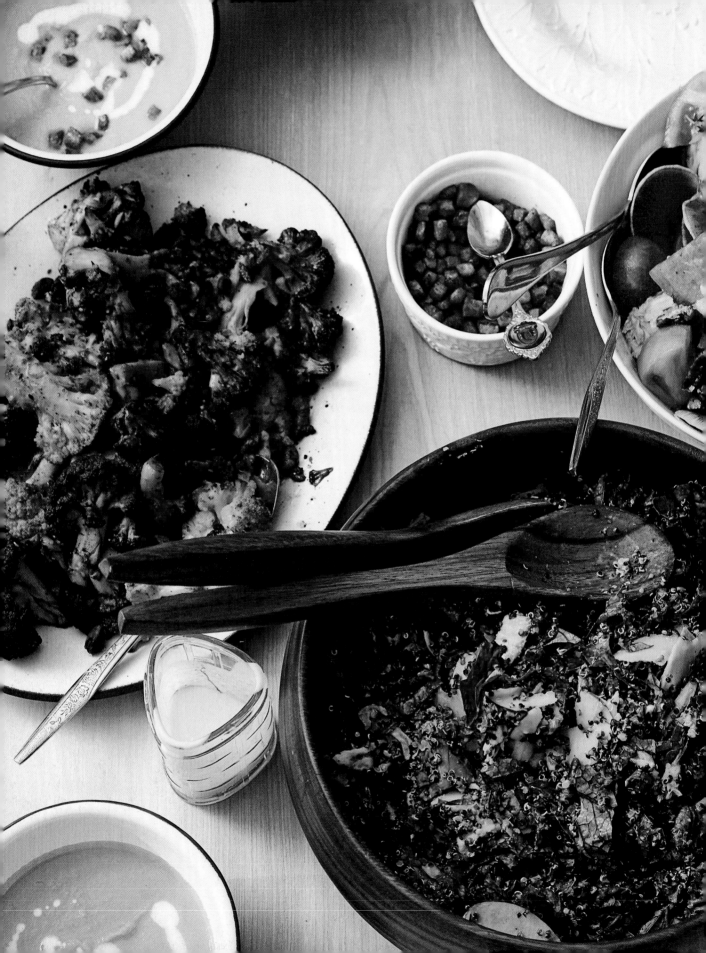

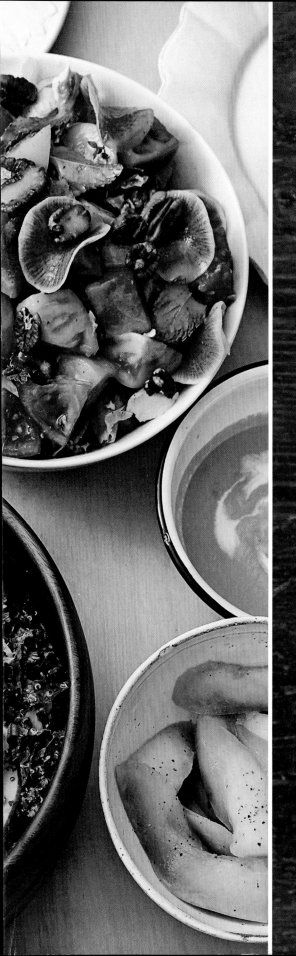

REAL FOOD HEALS

Eat to Feel Younger + Stronger Every Day

SEAMUS MULLEN
WITH GENEVIEVE KO

AVERY
an imprint of Penguin Random House
New York

A

AVERY

an imprint of Penguin Random House LLC
375 Hudson Street
New York, New York 10014

Most Avery books are available at special quantity
discounts for bulk purchase for sales promotions,
premiums, fund-raising, and educational needs.
Special books or book excerpts also can be created to
fit specific needs. For details, write SpecialMarkets@
penguinrandomhouse.com.

Library of Congress Cataloging-in-Publication Data

Names: Mullen, Seamus, author. | Ko, Genevieve, author.
Title: Real food heals : eat to feel younger and stronger
    every day / Seamus Mullen with Genevieve Ko.
Description: New York : Avery, an imprint of Penguin
    Random House, [2017] | Includes bibliographical
    references and index.
Identifiers: LCCN 2017012317 (print) | LCCN 2017014645
    (ebook) | ISBN 9780735213869 (ebook) |
    ISBN 9780735213852 (hardback)
Subjects: LCSH: Nutrition. | Diet therapy. | Prehistoric
    peoples—Nutrition. | High-protein diet—Recipes.
BISAC: COOKING / Health & Healing / Weight Control. |
    HEALTH & FITNESS / Diets. | COOKING /
Health & Healing / Low Carbohydrate.
Classification: LCC RA784 (ebook) | LCC RA784 .M757 2017
    (print) | DDC 641.5/63—dc23
LC record available at https://lccn.loc.gov/2017012317
p.   cm.

Printed in the United States of America
10 9 8 7 6 5 4 3 2 1

Book design by Ashley Tucker

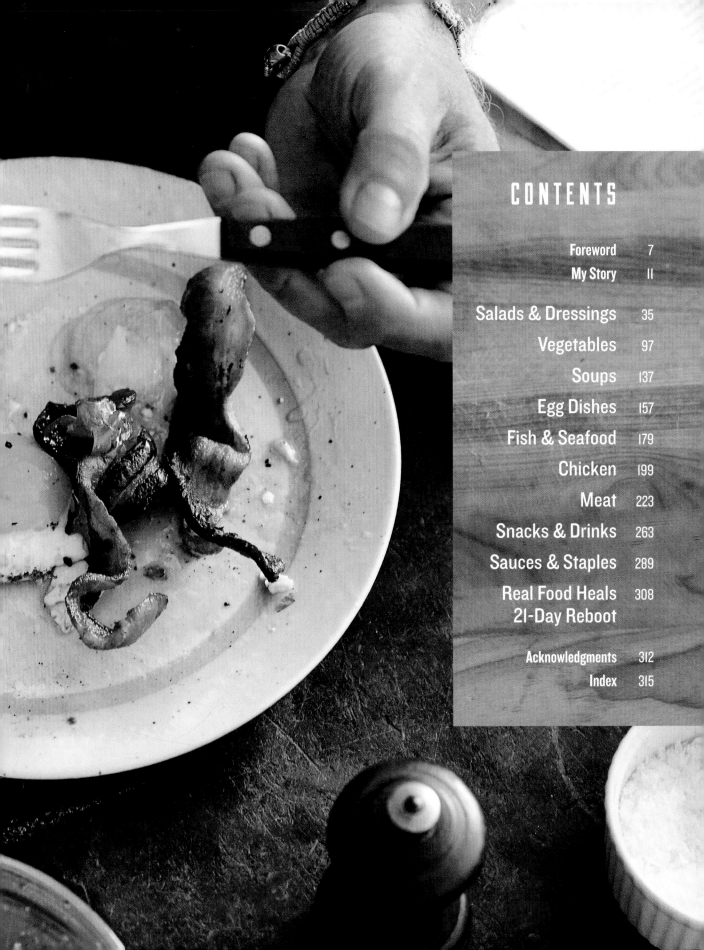

CONTENTS

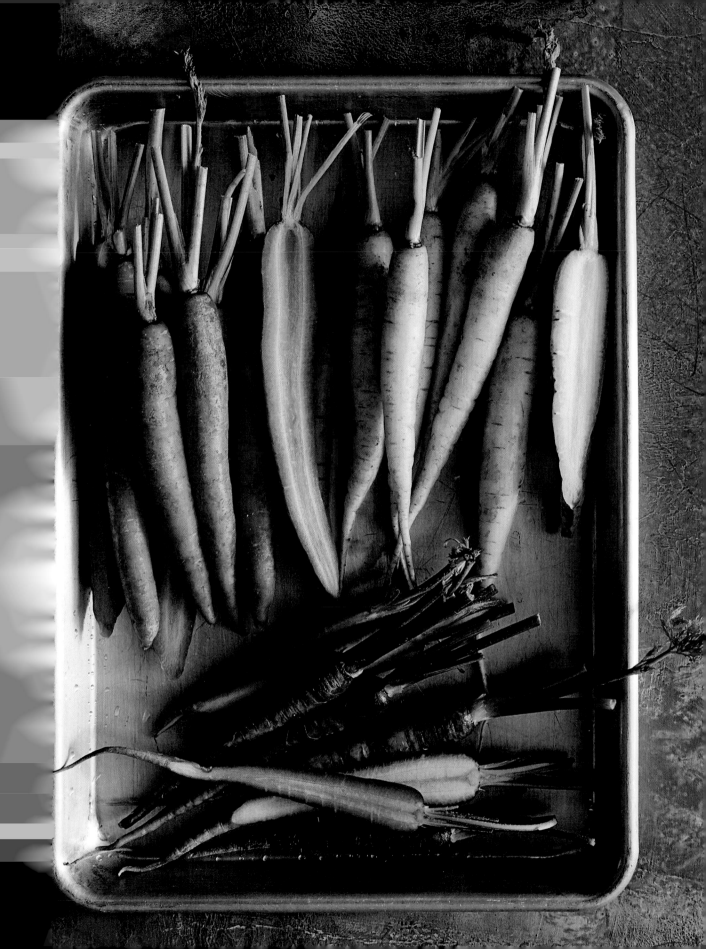

FOREWORD

In my practice as an integrative doctor, every day I meet and treat those who are unwell, from mildly so to very, very sick. When I met Seamus, he was firmly in the latter camp—the physical definition of what some might call "a hot mess." Professionally though, he was at the top of the New York chef food chain, cooking and running two successful restaurants, despite being profoundly unwell.

Though just in his thirties, he was struggling with the "older person's disease" of rheumatoid arthritis. He was in constant pain and drugged to the gills. He was carrying about fifty pounds of extra weight. He looked and felt awful and had been in this state for more than a decade. Worse, he wasn't getting well despite following all the recommended treatment protocols to the letter. After years of treatment, pain pills, anti-inflammatory drugs, and several near-death scares, Seamus had had enough. He knew there had to be another way. He had to get well, he just didn't quite know how that was going to happen.

When Seamus found his way to my office and shared his story, there was pain written all over his face. But it was his indomitable spirit that made the biggest impression on me. I knew that inside this very sick guy was a well one. We just had to find him.

In that first meeting, I remember telling Seamus that together we were going to make him feel better. How much better, I couldn't say, but we would do everything possible to push him toward wellness. We weren't going to mask the symptoms or dull the pain with more drugs, we were going to jump-start the healing process with one of the most powerful wellness-makers I know, the best medicine of all—food. The challenge? Seamus would need to change his relationship with it, top to bottom and forever. A tall order for some people, but not Seamus. He'd come to the end of the line (or was it the start?)—and he was ready to change everything. Seamus was all in.

As a chef, Seamus loved food and was surrounded by it, literally up to his elbows in it every day. Though he was in the business of nourishing others, he hadn't focused on nourishing himself. Like most people, and particularly sick people who are busy trying to just survive the day, Seamus hadn't given much thought to what food could actually do for him. Food had the power to be a healing, health-promoting "pill" on his plate, one whose "side effects" for him would include less pain, less inflammation and, ultimately, wellness. There were foods that could heal and sustain him, that would change the course of his life. It was up to me to guide him, and up to Seamus to take the ball and run with it—and run with it he did!

Fueled by his love of food and desire to be the strongest, healthiest guy we both believed he could be, Seamus took the food as medicine idea further than any patient I've ever worked with. What started with a mission to heal Seamus's gut—that critical, initial first step I take with many of my patients—blossomed into a healing journey and, ultimately, a total health transformation. To guide and mentor Seamus through this turnaround has been an honor and a joy, not to mention the genesis of one of the great health bromances of the decade! To see this challenging, personal, and ultimately triumphal journey come to life on the pages of this book is a gift that he is uniquely qualified to give—he has lived every inch of it and he is giving to others the tools they need to create their own health journeys through deliciously prepared, healthy, whole foods. It's a bonus neither of us could have imagined way in those early days.

The advantage in working with Seamus was that he was not only highly motivated to get well but also remarkably well positioned to do so. As an accomplished, award-winning chef, he possessed the exact skill set needed to treat his gut, once he had a healing-foods road map. Over the course of nine months, I saw Seamus nearly every week—often twice a week—and we tweaked his treatment and tweaked his diet. Within a few months, there was dramatic improvement. Within a year, he was off all his medications and free of any of the symptoms of his disease.

Today, I see a man completely different from the sick, broken-down guy who walked into my office six years ago. He's the poster boy for healthy living—super-fit; full of energy; and free of the extra weight, pain, and drugs that were dragging him under. Much as I'd sometimes like to think I could take all the credit for his dramatic turnaround, I am just as proud to have merely played a role in it. Seamus did all the hard work: learning, healing, changing his relationship with foods, and treating his body with care and respect. The student has become the teacher, and this book is the culmination of the education, transformation, and healing wisdom he gained along the way.

I'm extremely proud of him as a patient, but even more proud to call him a close friend—and now my mentor and inspiration in the kitchen. In so many ways, he put my medical practice into his delicious kitchen practice. The result is this gorgeous book, a hands-on guide that shows us that eating for health and wellness is really a celebration of nature's bounty. So, enjoy everything it has to offer and be well!

Frank Lipman, MD

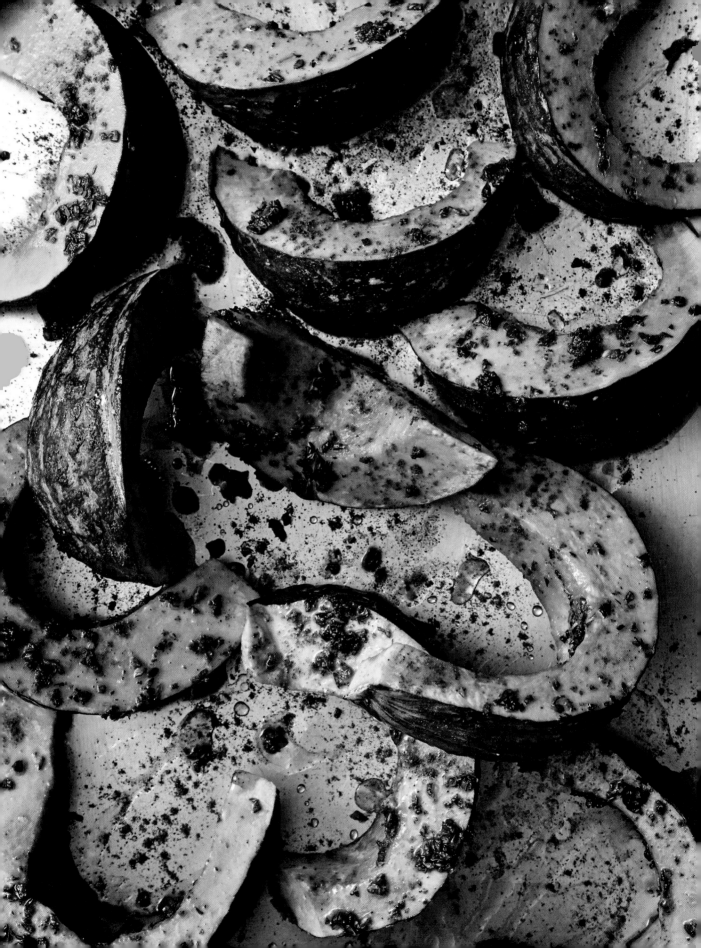

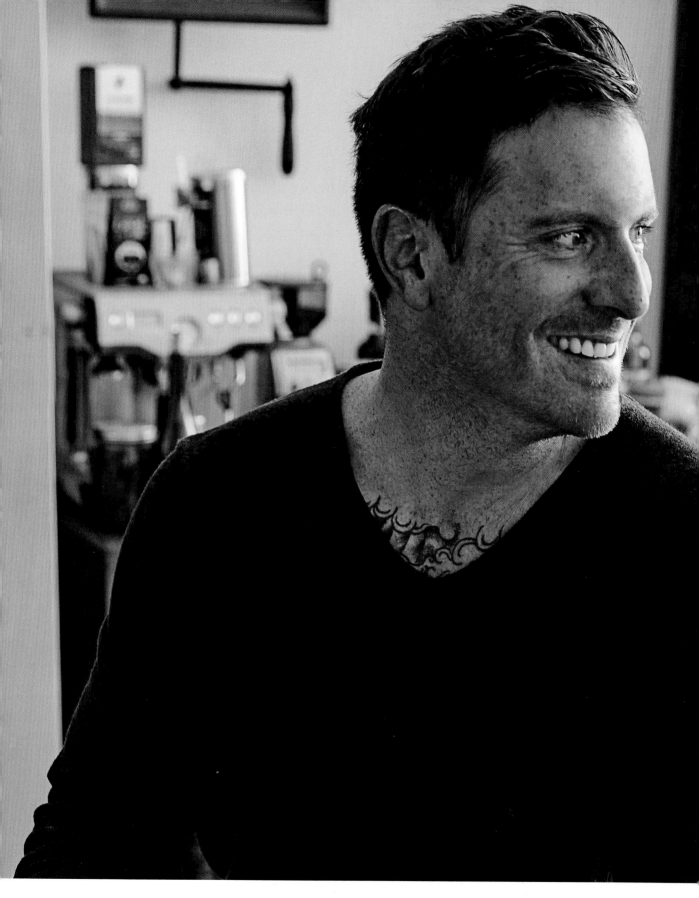

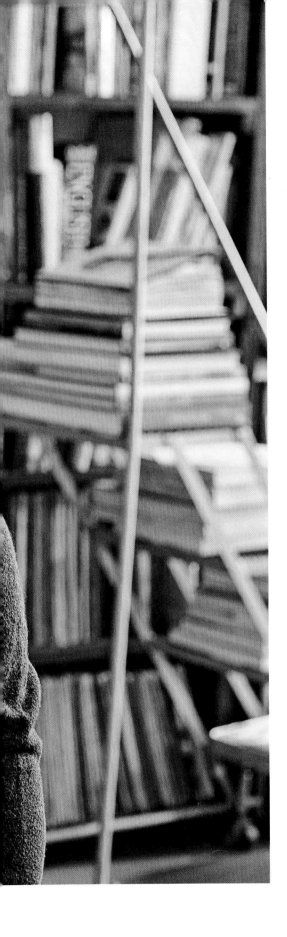

MY STORY

FOOD IS MY LIFE. IT MADE ME WHO I AM. IT NEARLY KILLED ME. AND IT SAVED ME.

I was born and raised on a farm in Vermont, where my parents and grandmother, whom I called Mutti, fed me freshly prepared whole ingredients. When I went to boarding school, I devolved into typical teenage boy behavior, shoveling junk food into my mouth. Even in college, when I began cooking seriously, I kept eating crap. Once I realized I wanted to be a chef, I started eating better, but my diet still revolved around carbs. Most of my professional training happened in Spain, where bread, rice, and noodles ruled my diet.

When I moved to New York City, I kept cooking and eventually opened two of my own restaurants, Tertulia and El Colmado, which I run today. As much as I loved cooking and the restaurant industry, I started to experience a lot of physical pain and my general health began to rapidly decline. Initially, I wrote off feeling like crap to the notoriously difficult life of the professional kitchen, but eventually it became clear that there was something seriously wrong with me and I needed help.

After several trips to the emergency room, I was finally diagnosed with rheumatoid arthritis (RA), a chronic inflammatory autoimmune disease. I struggled for years with RA, even while following the conventional treatment of disease management, and generally felt horrible. After a few years, I hit an all-time low. At the end of a day filming a food show, I could barely stand and felt feverish. I was being treated with immunosuppressant and anti-inflammatory drugs—as well as pain meds, to which I had become addicted—and I had gotten used to the severe flare-ups and awful side effects, but this time was different. I knew I needed to get to a hospital. By the time I arrived at the emergency room, my temperature had hit 106 degrees. The only thing that kept my brain from frying in the intensive care unit was plunging in and out of an ice bath.

I developed a cyclic headache so severe that I couldn't even see, and I slipped into unconsciousness. In that murky pain, I began to feel as if I were floating up in some sort of elevator shaft, and at the top of the shaft, a celestial sunlight glowed. I started drifting toward the light in this peaceful, effortless ascent. As I got closer to the light, I could feel that I was dying. In that moment, it would've been so easy to just give up and go into the light, but I told myself not to. I dug my fingers in and started pulling myself back down the shaft. As I got farther and farther away from the light, I started hearing beeping noises and voices, and eventually, I regained consciousness.

That's what it took for me to completely change my life, my diet, my fitness, and my overall well-being. Shit happens, and you can either get in the way of your body or you can get out of the way. I knew that something had to change or the next time this happened, I wouldn't survive. Through this experience, I began to learn the importance of being an active participant in my own well-being, and in doing so, for the first time in years I no longer felt helpless. Instead, I came to understand that the decisions I made directly affected the quality of my health. I sought out others who had gone through similar experiences and immersed myself in the world of Functional Medicine, which is an approach to health that addresses the root causes of illness rather than treating the symptoms of the illness, as is done in traditional medical practice. I met and became close friends with forward-thinking doctors, including Dr. Frank Lipman, and I realized that my poor health was directly linked to my carb- and sugar-driven diet.

I started exercising and eliminated gluten and grains, refined sugar, factory-farmed meat, and dairy from my diet, instead eating mainly vegetables and good proteins and fats. Over the past five years, I've fed my microbiome—the complex system of bacteria that lives in and on us—with foods that support a healthy and diverse population of bacteria, not with food-*like* substances that have a damaging effect on health. Not only have I avoided the emergency room, I've shocked doctors and everyone who knows me with my great health. At every checkup, the biomarkers of my disease are now non-existent. And I've experienced this incredible joy throughout the process, because my transformation has revolved around mindfully cooking and eating great food.

I want my experience to inspire you to live a fuller life through delicious food and 360 degrees of good health. I feel better than I ever have thanks to my new way of eating and living and want you to feel the same thrill—without having to suffer first the way I did.

In fact, my philosophy rejects any suffering, including the deprivation typical of diets, and champions joy in eating. My approach to nutrition starts with excellent food because I am, first and foremost, a chef. I want to change the way we eat with chef-quality dishes that are easy and fast enough to cook at home. I'm going to show you all the tricks of cooking like a chef—without the unnecessary fireworks—to give you the real value of streamlining your time in the kitchen.

For ten years, I worked, clawed, climbed, and finally dragged myself out of a pit of aches, pains, sickness, inflammation, broken bones, hospital visits, medications, countless hours in doctors' offices, and, most terrifying, two near-death experiences. With tremendous help from an amazing team of loved ones, colleagues, and doctors, the walls of this pit have gotten less and less slippery. And with a complete overhaul of my diet to one that celebrates vegetables, good fats, and proteins, and the joy of cooking and eating, I'm totally transformed, body and soul. Each day, I feel a little bit stronger, a little bit more complete.

This experience has been nothing short of a miracle for me. However, unlike miracles, which have neither rhyme nor reason, this change is the result of hard work, diligence, experimentation, and exhaustive research. In this book, I've put down what I've learned, from the recipes I've created in my home kitchen to the tips I've picked up from years of cooking and the guidelines I've adopted through research, work with doctors, and living a new life. I hope my food and my stories will not only inspire you to change but actually lead you to a new, delicious way of eating that makes you feel stronger, younger, and better every day.

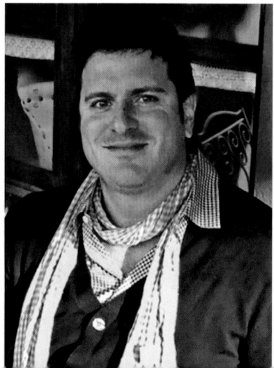
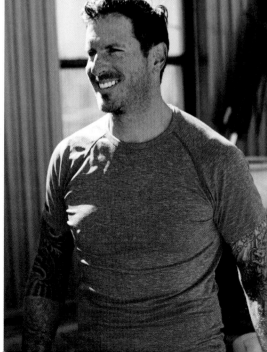

THE TENETS OF REAL FOOD HEALS

The only manageable and realistic way to maintain a lifetime of healthy choices comes from a positive and joyful relationship with delicious food. Follow these tenets and that's exactly what you'll experience.

PURSUE JOY IN THE KITCHEN. Cooking and eating are all about pleasure. Never lose sight of that priority.

NOTHING TASTES AS GOOD AS HEALTHY FEELS. It's important to draw the distinction between what may be enjoyable in the moment and what brings lasting joy. Choose the latter.

NUTRITIOUS FOOD IS DELICIOUS FOOD. How about a fresh ceviche of wild-caught seafood, avocado, pepitas, coconut, and lime? Delicious? Without question. Nutritious? Damn straight.

EAT REAL FOOD—as many vegetables and good fats and proteins as you want with meat and dairy as accents. Consume foods rich in probiotics and restrict carbohydrate and sugar intake.

COOK LIKE A PRO. Adhering to a few simple rules of the professional kitchen can help create incredibly dynamic, flavorful, exciting, and appealing dishes.

FORGET METRICS. Counting calories and tracking pounds gained and lost leads to the horrible antagonistic love-hate relationship with food that contributes to anxiety and low self-esteem.

EAT WHEN YOU'RE HUNGRY. We often eat on a schedule because we think we should. Transitioning from a carb-heavy diet to one of nutrient-dense vegetables, fats, and proteins means we eat less frequently and only when our bodies really need and want to.

BE PATIENT WITH THE CHANGE. It takes about a month to adjust from a carb-dependent diet to a vegetable-and-fat-based one. Stick to the tenets and wait for your body to switch from being a carb burner to being a fat burner. After that initial shift, the change is significant and lasting, and will make you feel stronger and

HOW TO USE THIS BOOK

Embracing a positive relationship with *real food* will change how you feel, improve your general health, and optimize your performance, regardless of what your baseline is. Whether your goal is to get off cholesterol medication, lose a few pounds, or reduce the symptoms of an autoimmune disease, learning to love foods that love you back is fundamental to achieving your goals.

I want you to use this book to reclaim your health. And I'm talking about 360 degrees of health. I want you to use these recipes together with exercise to reach a healthy body mass index, get good sleep, and feel happier. Along the way, you'll feel happier already as you learn that achieving sustainable health doesn't mean deprivation. These nutritious recipes are synonymous with *delicious* and will recalibrate what *delicious* means. Wherever you are in your journey toward wellness, you'll find what you need here. We are all unique, with unique nutritional needs, metabolisms, and goals, but the good news is that the broad strokes apply to everyone!

If you're already eating well, the recipes will give you new ideas for daily meals. If you generally eat well but slip up or overindulge occasionally, you'll find a range of dishes that are as indulgent and rich as any "cheat" food. If you're feeling bad physically and need a total transformation, start with the 21-Day Reboot (page 308) and go from there. Once you start eating this way, you're on the path to feeling your best and finding the sweet spot of where your body wants to be.

REDEFINING HEALTHY FOOD

It's time for us to redefine what constitutes healthy food. For too many years in America, what many have considered to be a healthy diet has actually been a formula for poor health. Take breakfast. The conventional wisdom has been that a healthy breakfast consists of a bran muffin, a juice, and a nonfat latte. This is simply one of the unhealthiest ways you can start your day.

This initial meal of sugar and carbohydrates sets up your metabolism for a roller coaster of sugar dependency that will last throughout the day. Just a few hours after breakfast, your energy sags and your hunger returns, causing you to reach for a midmorning snack before lunch. You'll probably grab another carb- and sugar-heavy snack, since that's what your body craves and what's most available. You'll get some relief, but only until lunch. That two-hour cycle of hunger keeps your blood sugar rising and falling all day long and keeps you eating nonstop. Even if you're consuming "low-calorie" meals and snacks, you end up eating a lot of total calories, few of which are beneficial.

This vicious cycle results in unnecessary cravings, fatigue, inflammation, mood swings, and weight gain.

So much of the advice we've been given to take control of our health has resulted in us getting sicker. *This has to change.*

The foods that provide the greatest health benefits and are the most satisfying are vegetables, good fats, and proteins. Those powerhouse staples form the foundation of how I cook and eat.

REMAKING HEALTHY FOOD

People often think healthy food is gross. Probably because much of so-called healthy food *is* gross! Plain steamed spinach doesn't exactly sing with flavor, but sauté it in olive oil, throw in some pine nuts and roasted garlic, and it's amazing! The other main problem with traditional "health" food is that it relies so heavily on the metrics of counting calories and fat grams. I believe that when making a lifestyle change, it's more important to consider the *quality* of calories than the quantity.

In these recipes, I stay away from all that fake garbage you see in diet books. You won't find gluten-free vegan grilled cheese or soy protein meat substitutes that are a poor attempt to remake unhealthy comfort food. Those substitutions often end up being unhealthier than the originals. They don't taste good, and they don't satisfy. Instead, I rely on lots of vegetables, good fats, and proteins, including a moderate amount of meat. A breakfast of scrambled eggs with mushrooms, okra, and bacon will keep you full until it's time for a lunch of kale salad with sardines, avocado, and herbs. That will keep you going until you sit down to a dinner of roasted squash and Brussels sprouts with pork chops. Not only are these types of food better for you, but they showcase the complex tastes and textures usually reserved for restaurant meals. You'll feel totally satisfied and happy eating truly healthy food.

A NOTE ON FATS

As my good friend Nina Teicholz, who wrote the incredible book *The Big Fat Surprise*, often says, "Fat is the most unfortunate homonym in the English language." What she means is that the word we use to refer to pesky belly fat is the same word we use to refer to cooking fats and fats we eat. About sixty years ago, it was theorized that since the fats we eat have more calories per gram than carbohydrates, they must be the driving cause of heart disease and obesity. It's not a stretch for people to imagine fats clogging our arteries. However, this is faulty and oversimplified science. Fats, and

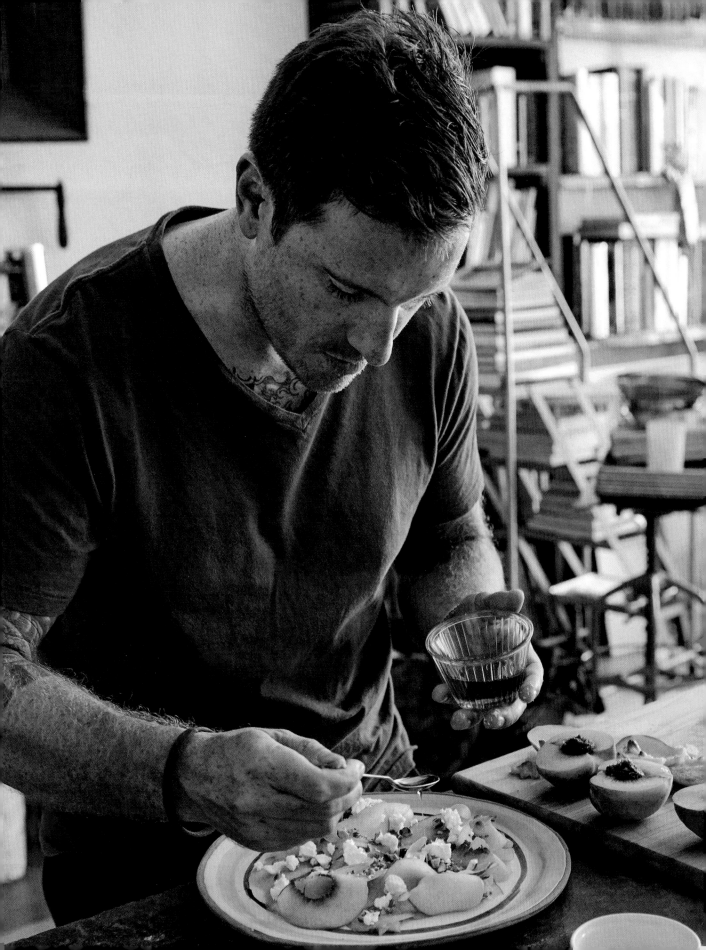

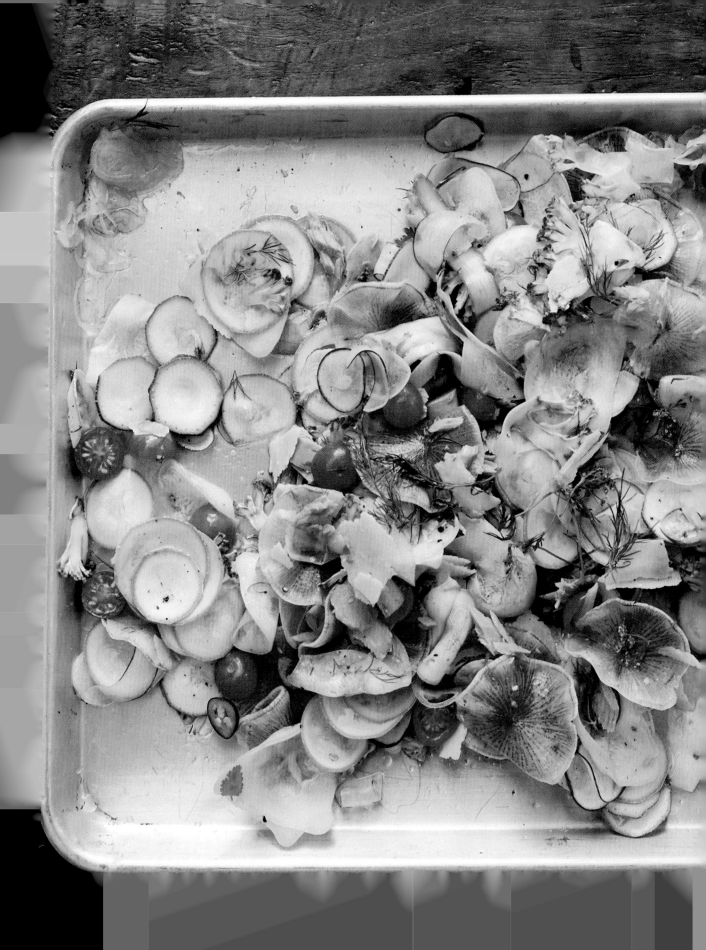

in particular saturated fats, have formed an essential part of the human diet for the entirety of our existence. When we started to fear fat and count calories is when our health as a nation really began to go off the rails. I only wish we had demonized refined sugar and not fats—then we might not have ended up in the pickle we're currently in. Fortunately, things are changing, and even the new federal dietary guidelines put greater emphasis on the importance of reducing refined sugar. Change is afoot, and I'm so excited food is driving that change.

UNDOING THE NOTION OF TRANSACTIONAL HEALTH

The first step to becoming a healthy person is believing you can be healthy. The day I stopped thinking of myself as a sick person was the last day I was a sick person. I believed I could get better, and that started me on my path to getting better. A crucial lesson I learned was to overcome what I call transactional health.

What does that mean? Well, transactional health is something that many of us are caught up in; it's a system of rewards and punishments, abstention and indulgence. Think calorie counting followed by cheat days. It's the idea that if you eat this pizza, you must go and work out and burn *x* number of calories to make up for it. To truly be healthy means to break up with the notion of transactional health, to walk away from an antagonistic relationship with food, to quit diets. I mean, after all, just look at the first three letters of the word *diet*.

When you embrace a positive relationship with *real* food, you can eat as much or as little as you want without feeling bad about the decision you've made and without any food remorse. Love the foods that love you back and you'll never need another "diet" again!

WHAT TO EAT

- **Unlimited amounts of vegetables and good fats.** Your body won't let you overeat these powerhouses. You can polish off supersize fries with ketchup, but you couldn't eat the same quantity of avocados. (Just avoid overeating nuts, especially roasted, salted ones.)

- **Meat and dairy in moderation.** Instead of using them as the main ingredients in a dish, treat them as you would seasonings, scattering some shaved Parmesan and some crumbled bacon over a salad.

- **If you're having carbs, choose sensible ones.** Limit yourself to vegetables and some fruits, wild or black rice, millet, and quinoa. If you're using grains, incorporate a small amount into a vegetable dish.

- **Get some good bugs in your body with probiotic-rich foods.** (More on the micro-biome below.)

- **Quality is always better than quantity.** There's a direct correlation between quality and quantity in food. The higher the quality, the lower the quantity you need to eat to feel satiated and happy.

GOOD BACTERIA FOR YOUR GUT

Feed your bugs. Trillions of microbes form our microbiome—an integral part of the immune system—and those little buggers are highly affected by the foods we eat. Eat plenty of prebiotic and probiotic foods to arm your body and help it fight off sickness.

- **Prebiotics:** Focus on fiber for prebiotic intake. The good bacteria in our guts likes fibrous, cruciferous vegetables, such as broccoli rabe, so I make sure to eat nutrient-dense veggies with every meal.

- **Probiotics:** Try at least a few bites of probiotics every day. Probiotics help cultivate a diversity of bacteria in us. They include fermented foods with living bacteria, such as sauerkraut and kefir.

WHAT TO AVOID

- **Limit sugar.** (More on that on page 22.)

- **Limit carbs.** Excessive carbohydrate consumption is toxic to our health. Eating more than 200 grams a day has a similar effect to eating too much refined sugar. It creates a metabolic roller coaster that requires us to eat more carbs to avoid hunger and fatigue.

- **Steer clear of convenience "food."** Processed food is designed to be craveable. It's very easy to effortlessly and mindlessly consume calories. We tend to eat junk far faster than we should, so our belly keeps demanding more before our brain gets the message that we've eaten enough.

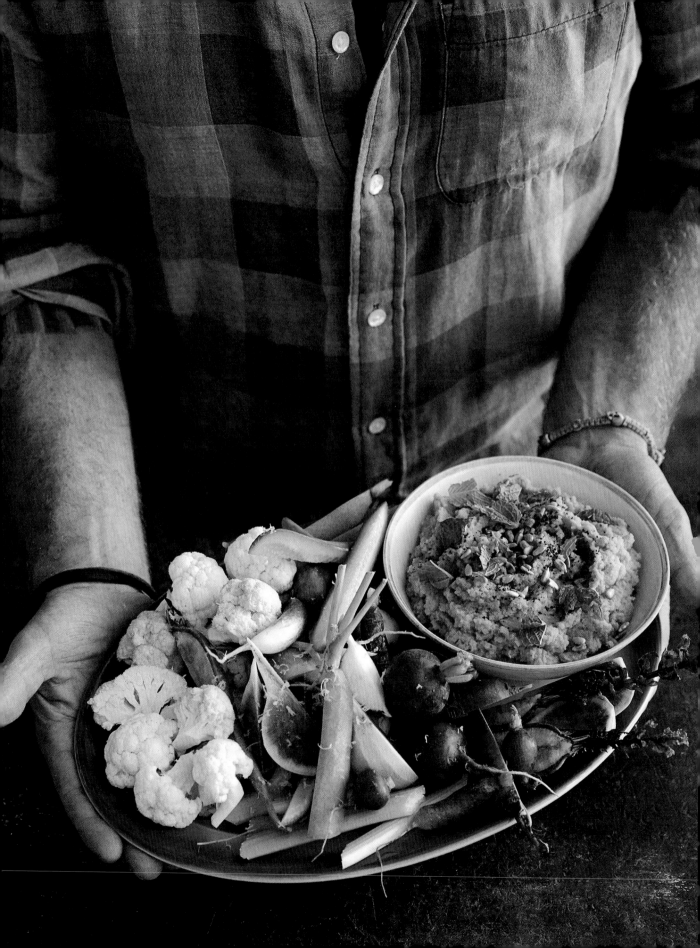

- **Stay away from overly processed foods.** Don't eat anything that is virtually unrecognizable from its original form, even when it comes to fresh foods. Choose a bunch of carrots over a bag of baby carrots, an apple over apple juice.

- **Avoid industrialized "vegetable" oils.** Highly oxidative oils like canola, corn, sunflower, and soybean oil are damaging to our cells and highly inflammatory. Instead, reach for oils like avocado, olive, ghee, and coconut, and saturated animal fats from pastured animals.

HOW TO EAT

- **Set aside time to eat proper meals, ideally with friends and family.** We so often take our meals slouching in couches, engaged with a device, or perhaps even driving, rather than around a table with our friends and families. If there is one consistent attribute of all cultures with many centenarians, it's the importance of socializing and joy, particularly around meal times.

- **Center the whole meal around vegetables.** Meat and dairy should be accents, if you eat them at all.

- **Try having lots of little plates instead of the conventional main dish with side dishes.** It takes the same amount of energy to prepare, and if you're doing lots of salads, it can be even quicker.

- **Savor the meal.** Eating slowly and taking breaks during the meal will give your body time to feel full.

- **Don't feel compelled to polish off leftovers.** If you're full and there's only a bite left, save it for the next day. There are no rewards for the clean plate club on this plan.

A SMARTER WAY WITH SUGAR

Sugar is the slippery and addictive slope to sickness. Unwanted excessive weight gain and the resulting risks for type 2 diabetes, hypertension, and general poor health are directly linked to overconsumption of sugar and the stress it puts on our bodies to produce insulin.

Sugar lurks in so many of our foods, especially readily available processed food-like substances. Sugar hides in breads, low-fat salad dressings, yogurts, and cereals, all of which, conventional wisdom has told us, are nutritious options. Drinks are especially dangerous. Fruit juices, sodas, and beer tend to have too much sugar without the benefit of any fiber. The sugar in those beverages hits our bloodstream fast and hard and has the ability to have an extremely deleterious impact on our health if they're part of our regular rotation.

But while I do suggest you avoid refined sugars as much as possible, natural sugar can be used—sparingly—to enhance good real foods. Maple syrup, honey, and fresh and dried fruits are healthier options, and you'll see I use them in my recipes.

We can all agree that everyone loves sugar. In fact, as part of human evolution, a love of sugar has been encoded in our DNA. But the refined sugar prevalent in modern food is extremely concentrated, a world away from less refined naturally occurring sugars. Make no mistake: Anything that ends in "–ose"—glucose, fructose, sucrose— is a form of sugar. As long as we're cognizant of that and consume it in moderation, we can enjoy it.

If given the choice, always reach for the least refined sugar that's closest to its natural state. Natural sugars have benefits to our health: Fresh and dried fruits have essential vitamins and fiber, raw honey has living bacteria that's good for the immune system, and pure maple syrup has antioxidants, magnesium, and enzymes.

From a flavor perspective, one of the great things about sweeter ingredients is that they temper and balance savory and acidic ingredients beautifully. Equilibrium is really important in a dish. In one moment, you want mouthwatering saltiness; in the next, you want to hit the taste buds with sweetness to balance it out. But you don't need a ton of sweetness. The less we overtax our taste buds with refined sugars, the more sensitive we become to sugars and the less we need to perceive it.

I also use sugar occasionally because it does what other ingredients can't: In a brine, pickling liquid, or salad dressing, it helps to temper the harsh acidity of vinegar. In a chicken marinade, it'll help the skin caramelize. With roasted vegetables, it brings forward their sweeter notes and browns them beautifully.

FINDING YOUR BODY'S RHYTHM

Our conventional-eating model—breakfast, lunch, and dinner with snacks in between— comes from a broken system of carb-dependency. The most important meal you have is the first meal, but that might be in the morning, or in the middle of the day, or in the afternoon. It should be a meal of vegetables, good fats, and proteins to keep you full longer without rises and dips in energy. Once you're able to recalibrate your metabolism and free yourself from a dependency on carbs and sugar to keep on an even keel, you'll find it's actually quite easy to go longer periods without eating. The benefits of that sort of intermittent fasting, not least of which is the hunger and excitement you'll feel when you eat a delicious meal to break that fast, are great.

I am staunchly against any sort of dieting or starvation for the sake of weight loss or for other emotionally driven reasons. But I think it's okay to feel hungry every once in a while. We are creatures of comfort, and in the modern world, we've gotten really bad at being uncomfortable. It gets a little too hot in the summer? Crank up the AC! Too cold in the winter? Crank up the heat! Hungry in the middle of the afternoon? Grab a sugar-laden "healthy" energy bar. What about enduring the discomfort for a little bit? I mean, we understand the importance of this with exercise, right? It's good to feel a little hungry from time to time. The important thing is to resist snacking and instead, eat a good, balanced meal of vegetables and protein and fats that is delicious and satisfying.

Once you stick to that type of eating, you'll discover your body's natural eating rhythm. I've found that I prefer to have my first meal around noon. I have vegetable-based soup and salad, maybe with a fried egg or a seared meat patty or fish fillet on top. It's delicious, hearty, and will keep me going until an early, lighter dinner with less meat and even more vegetables. I don't need to eat again until noon the next day. It may not be when I'm "supposed" to eat, but it's right for me and leaves me more energized. Find your rhythm and you'll feel healthier and happier.

CRAVINGS

How great would it be if the thing you craved the most was something that's so good for you? And I'm talking about a true craving, the kind your body—not your mind—wants.

The idea of a craving has come to mean that you want something you shouldn't. That illicit feeling makes you feel so good the moment the food touches your mouth. And modern food's screwed up because it's designed to do that. Tater tots with ketchup taste great for four seconds, but by the time you're done polishing off the plate, they're not amazing at all. You feel gross, you have food guilt, and you get down on yourself, asking, "Why did I do that?" You're just setting yourself up for disappointment. And the power of that food is that you don't even remember how bad it makes you feel. The next time you see it, you crave it again.

If you change the way you eat, from a carb-based diet to a vegetable-centric one, your body won't want what it used to. My body doesn't crave potato chips anymore. That doesn't mean I don't want to eat them. In my mind, I do. But I just don't crave

HOW TO RESIST TEMPTATION

Changing what your body craves is a process. Keep these points in mind when you're faced with temptation.

- **Be present when thinking about the foods you're consuming.** Rather than mindlessly eat, be thoughtful about what you're eating and whether it will leave you feeling good.

- **Identify your weaknesses.** Be aware of what tempts you most going into this change. I knew I couldn't resist salt-and-vinegar chips and sesame sticks, so I made sure I wasn't anywhere near them.

- **No cheat days.** You want your body to start seeking fat—not carbs—as a fuel source. You will be tempted during the shift. If you're dabbling in carbs during the transition, your body will burn them and want more of them.

- **After the transition, aim for moderation.** All the food in this book is delicious and indulgent, but there may be some favorites that aren't part of the plan. Allow yourself a little of something you love when sharing it with people you love.

- **Savor wine as a way of enjoying life.** If you're not in the process of a complete transformation or reboot, you can have a glass of wine when you're having a good time with friends or family. As with everything else you take in, be mindful of how much you're having and be sure that your intention is to share the experience with others, not to get drunk.

- **Only have dessert when it's worth it.** There are no desserts in this book because I believe you should avoid refined sugar. But if sweets are really important to you, then you should enjoy them occasionally as a treat. Be aware of how much sugar you're consuming and adjust everything you're taking in accordingly.

them anymore. Before I changed, I couldn't walk by salt-and-vinegar chips in the store without buying them. Now I see them and I know they're delicious, but I can walk past them with no regrets.

Here are the things I crave now: grilled avocado with blood orange; really good sashimi; ceviche; grilled asparagus with egg and Iberico ham; bacon; roast chicken; mushrooms. There's zero guilt associated with those cravings. I've gotten rid of my antagonistic love-hate relationship with food. I used to kind of hate myself for giving into late-night pizza cravings. Now I totally satisfy my cravings and feel great in every way.

COOKING TENETS
OF REAL FOOD HEALS

Cooking as a means of healing
makes the process more enjoyable.

Cooking nutritious food is not more restrictive.
It's more creative.

Cooking is about expression and improvisation.

Cooking is a craft, not an artistic endeavor.
It's not about ego or performance. It's not about
impressing people to inflate your own sense of self-worth.

Cooking is about making nourishing food.

Cooking is about soul.

Cook from the heart, cook for the body,
cook with love.

KITCHEN GUIDELINES

When I help people look at how they cook and eat and how they might make some positive changes in their relationship with food, I try to stay away from hard and fast *rules*. Instead, I just help set up some structure. After all, we're all very different and what works for one person may not work for the next. That said, there are some basic tenets I like to follow whenever I'm planning and prepping my meals.

- **Make food delicious.** When cooking becomes a task no less utilitarian than putting on a raincoat when it's raining, you're in trouble. Food is meant to be pleasurable. Along with sex, it's one of the most indulgent things we can experience. Take a few minutes to put some extra love into your cooking and the result will pay dividends on your health.

- **Consider the origins of your food.** If you can't pronounce it, you probably don't want to cook with it. I know this sounds pretty basic, but when you're looking at a label, think about what the ingredients are. If you've never heard of them before or they don't sound like food, it's best to stay away.

- **Make cooking quality time.** We can't overlook the health value of stopping our busy lives and cooking and eating together, engaging with other humans. Let's not forget how important it is to break (gluten-free!) bread with others.

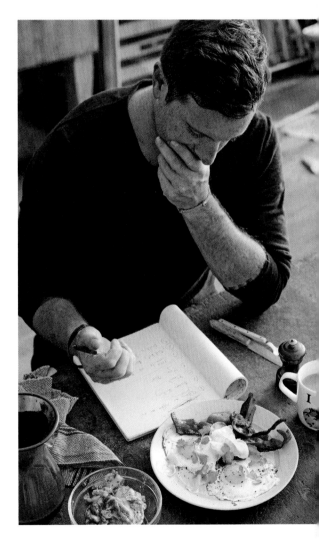

CHEF TIPS FOR MAKING HEALTHY FOOD DELICIOUS

I'm a firm believer that first and foremost, food needs to be delicious. There is simply nothing very inspiring about a bland bowl of flavorless quinoa. Yeah, perhaps it might be "healthy," but who really wants to eat it? Where is the joy? Where is the pleasure?

As a professional chef, I've watched from a distance as the Internet has exploded with endless recipes for healthy food. And while there are a lot of great ideas and great dishes circulating, I find that the little tricks of the trade that we chefs learn growing up in professional kitchens are often overlooked. Armed with a little bit of savvy and a well-tuned palate, you can turn the ordinary into the extraordinary.

- **Season, season, season.** One of the most common mistakes home cooks make is not being assertive enough when it comes to seasoning. Often, a little extra salt and pepper or even some lightly chopped herbs will go a long way toward bringing out the natural flavors of a dish. Just imagine a roast chicken without salt and pepper. Blech! Now add some coarse sea salt, cracked pepper, crushed thyme and rosemary, lemon zest, maybe even some coriander seeds and sesame seeds. Suddenly, that pedestrian bird has become a flavorful masterpiece.

- **Season as you go.** You want to add salt in stages to build flavor. Taste your salt to see how salty it is and adjust the amounts you add to your dish accordingly. Keep in mind that teaspoon for teaspoon, finer salts tend to add more saltiness.

- **Start with good salt.** I prefer sea salt for its complex and concentrated saltiness and its abundance of minerals. My friends at Jacobsen Salt Co., in Portland, Oregon, harvest all their salt from the pristine waters of the northwestern coastline. I often finish dishes with Jacobsen's flake finishing sea salt and really like Jacobsen's specialty salts, particularly the one infused with ghost chile.

- **Think of the four points of the compass of our palate: salty, sweet, sour, spicy.** Playing spicy off sweet (think: mango and chiles) or sour off salty (think: salt-and-vinegar chips) can make a dish really feel balanced and craveable. I don't always have these elements in equal parts. Sometimes you want one flavor profile to dominate the others, but having a balance makes for a successful and exciting dish.

- **Food tastes better when it looks good.** I'm not saying you should pull out tweezers to compose fussy plates of food, but you shouldn't dump the food on a plate. There's a difference between rustic and sloppy.

- **Finish dishes with soft herbs.** They're really healthy, add a bright pop, and change the character of a dish to make it tastier and more exciting. I add them at the end so they stay bright. Feel free to use whatever you like or have on hand. To chop them, I run a knife through them just enough to discipline them, or I simply tear them up by hand.

MOTIVATION TO MOVE

I know it's hard to exercise regularly—to find the time, energy, and will to do it. But you have to. It's the difference between living and dying. Food plays a huge role in how your body functions, but movement does, too. I don't know what will motivate you to get moving, but here's what did it for me.

While recovering from health scares and overhauling my diet, I decided to return to cycling competitively. And I decided I needed a goal, something to push toward. I thought of the most difficult physical challenge I could that might still be within my reach, and I decided to compete in La Ruta de Los Conquistadores in 2014.

La Ruta is touted as the most difficult mountain bike race in the world. I'm not sure if you can quantify that sort of thing, but from what I've seen—and now experienced firsthand—it's pretty damn hard. It's a three-day race, going from the Pacific coast of Costa Rica to the Atlantic, covering 161 miles and 29,000 feet of vertical climbing over five mountain ranges. All off road.

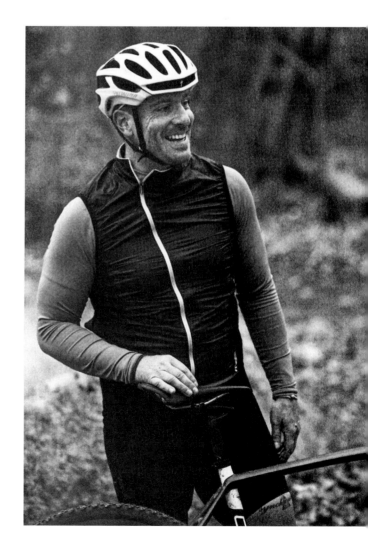

My training involved working out five or six times a week, lowering my body fat, dropping weight, getting stronger, and teaching my muscles how to endure suffering and then recover as quickly as possible so that they could go right back to suffering again.

During one workout in Prospect Park in Brooklyn, I was riding alone, pushing really hard, and feeling strong on the bike. After passing a peloton of strong riders, spinning hard at 26 mph, I heard heavy breathing from behind me, followed by a raspy voice with a West Indian accent egging me on: "Come on, man! Work it out,

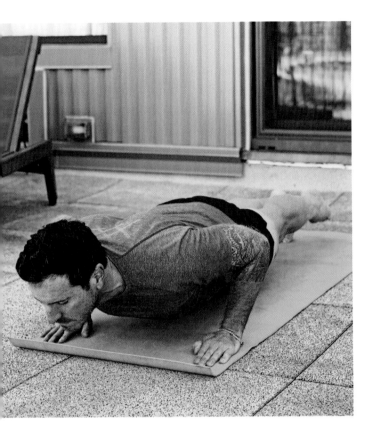

you got it, push it, bring it!" At first, I was annoyed that this guy behind me was sucking my wheel and pushing me to work harder so he could draft me and benefit from my hard pull. But when I looked over my shoulder, I saw the elated face of a guy who looked to be in his fifties, with a graying goatee, sweat and salt caked on his face, pushing hard to push me harder. I was inspired.

He was riding a gorgeous and very, very expensive bike, and the joy on his face was infectious. As we approached a big descent, he kept pushing me to pedal harder—I did, and we ripped past a second group of strong riders, now pushing 40 mph, his front wheel glued to my back wheel. We came into the straightaway and continued to push a hard gear, maintaining our speed. Toward the end of the flats, he pulled by me, slapped my ass, and said, "Good work. See you next time!" As he peeled off and left the park, I noticed something strange about him, and it took me a minute to realize that where his left leg should have been, he had a prosthetic leg from the knee down, fitted into his bike shoe, clipped to his pedal. Whoa. Not only was he many years my senior, but he had only one leg!

I hope to see him in the park and ride with him again, but if I don't, I won't ever forget him pushing me on from behind, encouraging me. He obviously had no idea how much I had to overcome to get to where I was on the bike, but seeing him and all that he had to overcome to get to where *he* was made me realize one thing: no excuses.

A VAIN—AND VALID—REASON TO EXERCISE

You should feel good about your body. Feeling young and strong is amazing—and something I wish I'd discovered earlier. When I see myself naked, I'm proud of what I see. I couldn't say that even a few years ago—or any years before that, for that matter. It's not that I'm an Adonis now, but I'm over a lifetime of self-loathing, because I know that exercising and eating well all the time make my body the best that it can be. I finally know what it feels like to feel good. There's a breakthrough moment that has to happen if you've never arrived at this stage of self-love, and it has to start by getting up and moving.

HOW TO CHANGE YOUR BODY THROUGH MOVEMENT

My mantra tends to be "Use it or lose it!" It's 1 percent theory, 99 percent practice. This goes for a lot of things, but I think of it in terms of the body. The human body is really good at doing whatever you do a lot of. If you do a lot of sitting around eating potato chips, it gets really good at sitting around and eating potato chips. If you do a lot of moving and laughing, it gets good at moving and laughing.

Establishing a positive relationship with real food will motivate you to move. The more you move, the more you'll crave real food. One positive behavior enforces the other. As with all things in life, success lies in balance. Balancing healthy stress in physical exertion with nutrition and recovery is an integral step to reclaiming your health.

MOVE intentionally.

EAT mindfully.

REST thoroughly.

Cycle those three steps and you will slow the degeneration that comes with aging and subpar health.

HOPE FOR ME, HOPE FOR YOU

In my mid-thirties, I was sick and getting sicker. I could barely get out of bed in the morning, and my baseline was chronic pain which frequently cascaded into extreme suffering. I knew there had to be another way to approach my illness, and I was unwilling to let my declining health ruin my life. So I threw myself into learning as much as I could about the forward-thinking practice of Functional Medicine, which aims to address the root causes of illness rather than focus on symptomatic treatment.

I read remarkable stories about people who had reversed chronic "incurable" autoimmune diseases like Crohn's disease and multiple sclerosis (MS). I watched countless TED Talks. I consumed Pub Med reports on the impact of diet on autoimmune disease,

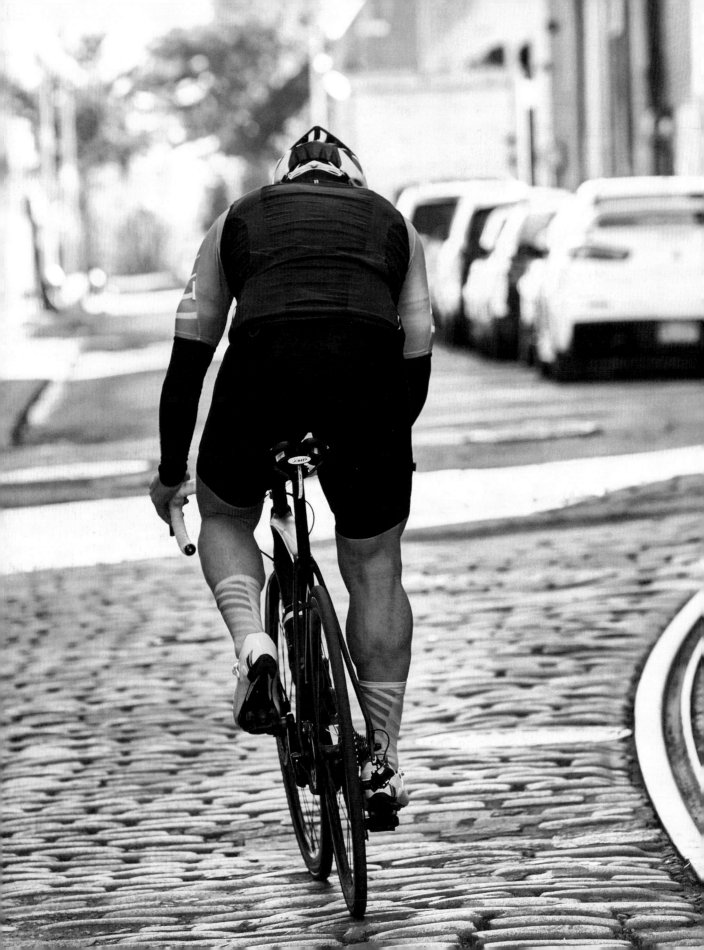

and one day, I stumbled upon a podcast by the remarkable Dr. Terry Wahls. Terry is a clinical professor of medicine who was living with severe, progressive MS. Through the development of a modern-day hunter-gatherer diet, Terry went from using a reclining motorized wheelchair to riding a bicycle in six months. I also met and became close friends with Ari Meisel, a young professional who reversed his Crohn's disease, got off all his medications, and went on to compete in Ironman triathalons.

Their stories inspired me, motivated me, and made me believe that one day I would be able to join them in telling my own story of success. I realized that these were not superhuman anomalies, but everyday people like me who were suffering and had had enough of being sick. What they had in common was tenacity, a characteristic that I pride myself on having as well. I knew that if they could do it, I could too. And that began my path out of the darkness of physical hell and into the light of wellness.

I now know that nutrient-dense plants like mustard greens, kale, cabbage, asparagus, blueberries, and rhubarb; nourishing fats and proteins like wild fish, nuts, and seeds; and sustainably raised meats are the building blocks of health. And it just so happens that with a little thought and a few tricks and techniques, they are the most incredibly delicious ingredients to eat!

When I was sick, my initial goal was simply to feel a little better, perhaps increase my overall health a bit, do *something* to not feel so helpless. I never could have imagined the sort of success I was about to experience. Within six months, I was riding a bicycle again. Within a year, I was off my powerful medications and symptom-free.

Once I got a taste for feeling strong, all I wanted was more. I decided that it wasn't enough just to *overcome* an incurable disease—I wanted to be so strong that *no disease* would stand a chance against me. I know that embracing a positive relationship with food and celebrating *real foods every day* makes us so strong that disease doesn't stand a chance. Sure, there will be colds and flus (but far less frequently!) and bumps and bruises along the way, but our probability for developing a chronic disease drops dramatically when our general health is strong. And to be strong means to embrace 360 degrees of wellness 365 days a year. If you do this, you will become the best expression of yourself. This is my promise to you.

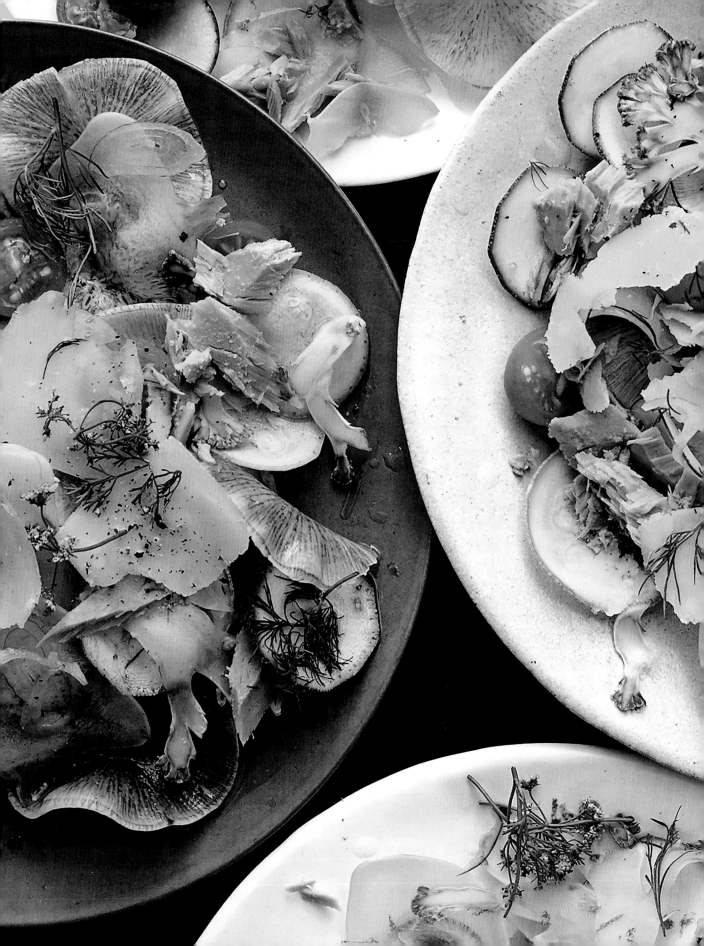

SALADS & DRESSINGS

Salads may be my favorite thing to eat. They're a riot of colors, textures, and tastes. I see no reason why salads should be limited to lettuce, so I've composed salads with all types of vegetables that are available throughout the year. Each vegetable combination is paired with a dressing designed just for it, but you can easily mix and match to your taste. There are just a few things to remember when you want to build a really delicious salad:

- No brainer, but start with the best possible vegetables. Get them from your garden or a local farmer and, if possible, buy organically grown produce.

- When I'm composing salads, I find myself putting together elements that seem almost architectural. The shape of some ingredients, like radish rounds, is very geometric; others, like torn lettuce, are very organic. The result looks cool and eats well.

- Make the bulk of the salad vegetables. But feel free to mix types; use the same ones raw or cooked, or swap in something that looks good at the market.

- Make extra dressing. That way, you can have a salad any time.

- Use dairy as an accent. I really limit dairy, but sometimes, I use just a little bit to accentuate the great flavors and textures in a dish. I'd feel terrible if I ate fondue, but I feel fine—actually, even happier—when I throw a little crumbled or shaved cheese on a salad.

- Toss the dry vegetables and accompaniments together first. Sometimes I season with salt and pepper and toss again, then drizzle on the dressing and toss a final time. This ensures that the vegetables are mixed well, seasoned well, and evenly coated. If you add the dressing before the salt, you may end up with clumps of salt.

- Eat immediately. Some salads keep well, but most taste best right after they're dressed. If you want to pack a salad to go, just keep the dressing separate.

SALAD TOOLS

I toss salads with my hands, but rely on a few other tools to make them perfect.

- **Embrace the Microplane.** This tool is the best secret-flavor weapon in the kitchen arsenal. I think I use the Microplane more than any other kitchen tool, using it to grate horseradish, nuts, citrus, garlic, ginger, and turmeric. Originally developed as a woodworking tool, this ultra-fine rasp grater ended up being used by Italian chefs to grate hard aged Parmesan cheese. As it turns out, there are a million and one other applications for the Microplane in the kitchen. My favorite is to finish a dish by zesting citrus over it. A little lemon makes a salad come to life; lime gives a bright, floral, and unexpected tropical jolt of flavor; and grapefruit and orange taste brilliant. Imagine a roasted beet salad with grapefruit segments, pistachios, and a little grapefruit zest as a garnish. The most important thing to remember when zesting citrus is to start with organic fruit and always wash the fruit well.

- **You need a big-ass bowl.** It's much easier to toss a salad when there's enough room for the vegetables to move.

- **When it comes to making vinaigrettes,** I use the Microplane to grate in a little garlic. I want just enough to get the delicate flavor and essential oils of garlic, which are important for feeding a healthy microbiome. I like how the Microplane lets the garlic melt into a vinaigrette or into gently steamed or sautéed vegetables without overpowering the dish the way chopped garlic can.

- **Get a mandoline.** You don't have to splurge on the fancy French kind. The little Japanese benriner works amazingly well. (Be sure to watch your fingers, though!) If you don't have one, you can't cut paper-thin slices very easily. If you're in the market for a food processor, the Breville Sous Chef is my favorite, as it has an adjustable mandoline attachment that makes slicing raw vegetables easy and safe.

- **Use a glass jar with a lid to make the dressing.** Most of my dressings combine all the ingredients in a jar to be shaken until emulsified. Whatever's left over can be kept in that jar and shaken again whenever you're ready for another salad.

If you have green, unripe avocados that you want to eat now, make this dish. I first created it when I was traveling in Pantelleria, a tiny Italian island off the coast of Tunisia. One morning at the local market, I found a ton of underripe green avocados. I was craving avocado, but too impatient to wait for them to ripen. It dawned on me that the hard fruits were perfect for slicing on a mandoline. The technique gives avocado a melt-in-your-mouth texture. Those buttery slices bring together the sweetness of cherries with the saltiness of smoked salmon. The trio of avocado, salmon, and walnuts packs this with good fats that will keep you satisfied.

SERVES 2

AVOCADO CARPACCIO WITH SMOKED SALMON, WALNUTS, AND CHERRIES

I green avocado, halved, pitted, and peeled

Jacobsen flake finishing sea salt

Walnut oil or extra-virgin olive oil

6 Rainier cherries, pitted and chopped

I ounce smoked salmon, torn

2 tablespoons Buttered Salted Walnuts (page 304)

Fresh mint leaves

Slice the avocado on a mandoline into very thin slices directly onto a serving plate. Sprinkle with salt, then drizzle with walnut oil. Scatter the cherries all over, then drape the salmon on top.

Break the walnuts over the dish, then tear the mint leaves and scatter them over the top. Serve immediately.

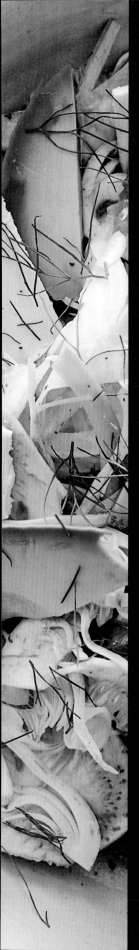

ARTICHOKES

Artichokes are the poet warriors of the vegetable kingdom: They have these prickly exteriors, but tender hearts, like sensitive soldiers in plate armor. It's remarkable that we eat the leaves at all, given the battle involved in getting to the tasty parts. The first person who ate an artichoke must've been insanely hungry. I'm glad that adventurous eater did, though, because the heart's grassy freshness and succulence is delicious. Plus, it is one of the ideal foods for feeding *Bacteroides fragilis*, the family of healthy bacteria in our gut's microbiome.

HOW TO PREP ARTICHOKES

Cut a lemon in half, squeeze the halves into a medium bowl, and drop in the rinds (this is your acidulated water). Add cold water to a depth of 4 inches or so. Pull the rough outer leaves off the artichoke. You do this first step by hand because you have more control that way. Turn the artichoke upside down and cut off all the dark green leaves with a sharp paring knife, turning the artichoke in your hand while you slice with the other. Turn it right side up, trim the stem to I inch, and run the knife up the stalk to remove all the darker green peel around the stem. As you cut, keep dipping the artichoke and knife in the acidulated water to prevent oxidation. Cut off and discard the purple flower at the top, then scrape out the furry choke in the center. Keep the prepped heart in the acidulated water while you work on the rest of the artichokes you're going to use.

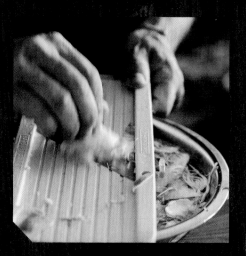

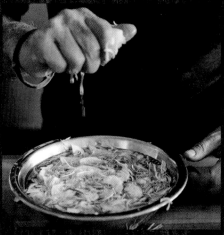

This salad makes me so happy. There's no sacrifice of flavor with this dish—or with the way I eat generally. Olive oil is so nice with artichoke and fennel, which get shaved thin so you get their fresh crunch without aggressive fibrous toughness. To keep that delicate crispness, have the vinaigrette ready to go so the vegetables don't sit before getting dressed. I use just a little bit of ricotta salata for its nice crumbly-creamy texture. If you have pine nuts hanging around, toast them and toss them on top for another rich accent.

SERVES 2 TO 4

FENNEL AND ARTICHOKE SALAD WITH GRAPEFRUIT

I small fennel bulb

I large artichoke, prepped (see facing page)

¼ cup Lemon Dijon Vinaigrette (recipe follows), plus more to taste

I grapefruit

I avocado, pitted, peeled, and thinly sliced

I½ ounces ricotta salata, sliced and broken into shards

Jacobsen flake finishing sea salt and freshly ground black pepper

Pick off and reserve the fronds from the top of the fennel. Run the fennel bulb and stems on a mandoline to create paper-thin slices, then mandoline the artichoke heart as well. Toss the fennel and artichoke slices in a large bowl with the dressing to prevent oxidation.

Trim the top and bottom of the grapefruit, then use a paring knife to cut off all the pith and peel. Reserve the peels. Cut out the grapefruit segments between the membranes. Cut the segments into bite-size pieces and add to the bowl. Squeeze all the juice you can from the membranes into the bowl, then discard. Gently toss and add more dressing to taste.

RECIPE CONTINUES ▶

3   Divide the mixture among serving plates and top with the avocado and ricotta salata. Zest some of the reserved grapefruit peel on top, then sprinkle with the reserved fennel fronds. Season with salt and pepper and serve immediately.

LEMON DIJON VINAIGRETTE MAKES ABOUT ⅔ CUP

For an all-purpose dressing, I combine vinegar and lemon because the former is really tart, but with a little sweetness that lemon juice doesn't have. That sour duo is balanced by mellowing olive oil and the heat of mustard. I like using the Laurent du Clos whole-grain mustard here because I want some spiciness in the mix.

Zest and juice of 1 lemon

2 tablespoons champagne vinegar

1 tablespoon whole-grain Dijon mustard

¼ garlic clove, grated on a Microplane

⅓ cup extra-virgin olive oil

Jacobsen flake finishing sea salt and freshly ground black pepper

In a glass jar, combine the lemon zest and juice, vinegar, mustard, garlic, and oil with a large pinch of salt and a few grindings of pepper. Seal the jar tightly and shake well. Season with salt and pepper. Shake again just before serving.

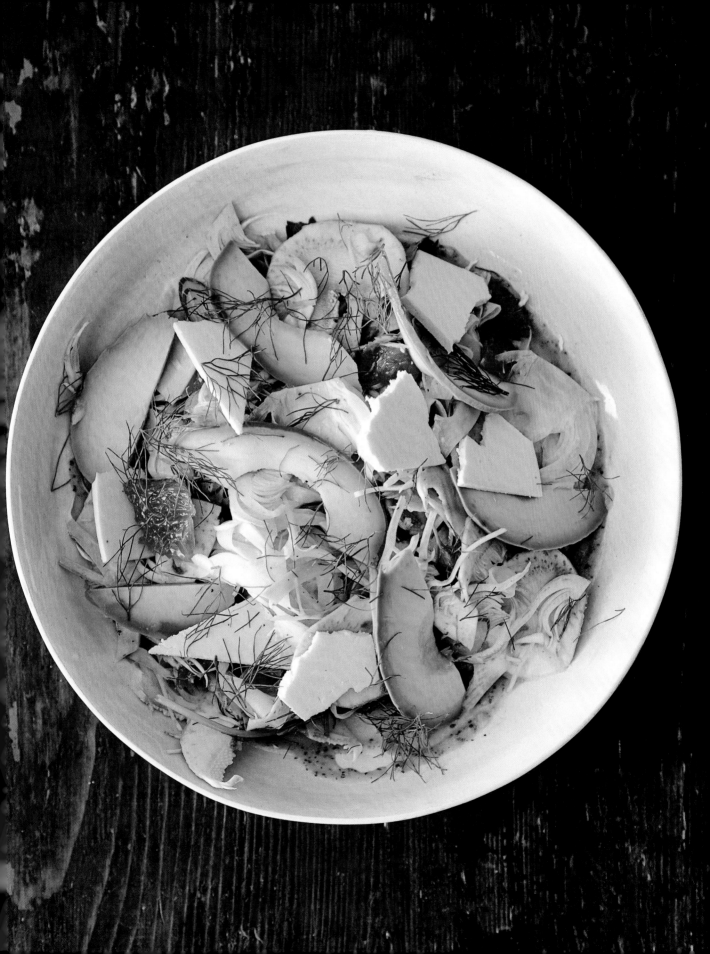

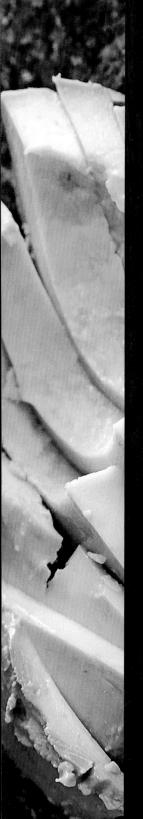

AVOCADOS

Avocados are experiencing an unprecedented moment of glory. Once upon a time, we mistakenly thought they were artery-clogging fatty fruit that should be avoided. Turns out, they're one of the healthiest foods we can eat. I couldn't be happier about their newfound celebrity. I am, after all, a chef who also happens to be a health and fitness advocate *and* an avocado freak.

There are literally hundreds of varieties of avocado, but the Hass, which is most commonly grown in Southern California, represents the lion's share of avocados on the American market.

So the obvious question is, how can there be hundreds of varieties of avocado and only one popular dish made with them? I'm here to show you there's so much more to avocados than guacamole. Here are a few of my favorite ways to use them.

- **Smoothie:** My day nearly always starts with avocado. Just cutting into the fruit and seeing that gorgeous pastel yellow-green puts a smile on my face. The easiest way to get that goodness into your gut is to use it as a creamy base for your green smoothie. I'll toss avocado, kale, ginger, banana, honey, and unsweetened coconut water in the blender for a silky-smooth, filling breakfast.

- **Toast:** This is a modern classic. I don't eat gluten, so rather than bread, I make "toast" with toasted nori. I top it with avocado slices, a few thin slivers of jalapeño, a squeeze of lime, a few sprigs of cilantro, and a sprinkle of crunchy sea salt. You can also add some radish or radish sprouts or even some excellent canned tuna in olive oil.

- **Salad:** My take is super simple. I drizzle avocado chunks and hearts of palm with coconut oil and lime juice, then top them with a little cilantro, mint, basil, and thinly sliced shallots.

- **Vinaigrette:** To amp up a simple salad, I blend an avocado, a clove of garlic, some lemon or lime juice, a little full-fat organic kefir, and some green herbs like basil or tarragon until smooth. Then I blend in some olive oil and season with salt and pepper. I toss the creamy dressing with butter lettuce, some herbs, cherry tomatoes, and some sunflower seeds or nuts.

- **Eggs:** Scrambled eggs with avocado are a favorite—and not just for breakfast. I sauté some vegetables—maybe some shallot rings, summer squash chunks, green beans—in olive oil over low heat. Then I add beaten eggs and gently fold them together. When they are nearly set but still a little wet, I add diced avocado. For a supercharged meal, whisk a tablespoon of chia seeds into your eggs 5 minutes before cooking them.

- **Grilled:** I cut the skin-on fruit into halves or quarters and season with salt and pepper, then grill until grill marks appear and the fruit is warm. I serve the pieces with a sprinkle of Japanese togarashi spice blend, a squeeze of lemon, and some sea salt and sesame oil.

- **Soup:** This chilled soup is a delicious summery starter. Blend a few avocados, some garlic, kefir or coconut milk, cilantro, and coconut oil until smooth. Season with salt and pepper and chill. Serve cold (within a few hours) with some thin slices of serrano chiles, a drizzle of olive oil, and some cilantro leaves.

- **Cups:** I scoop the flesh out of the fruit, dice it, and toss it with some grapefruit, fresh herbs, olive oil, and salt, then toss it back into the skin. If you're into dairy, burrata or fresh mozzarella makes a decadent addition. It's the perfect little snack.

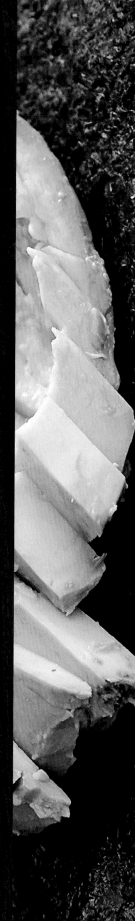

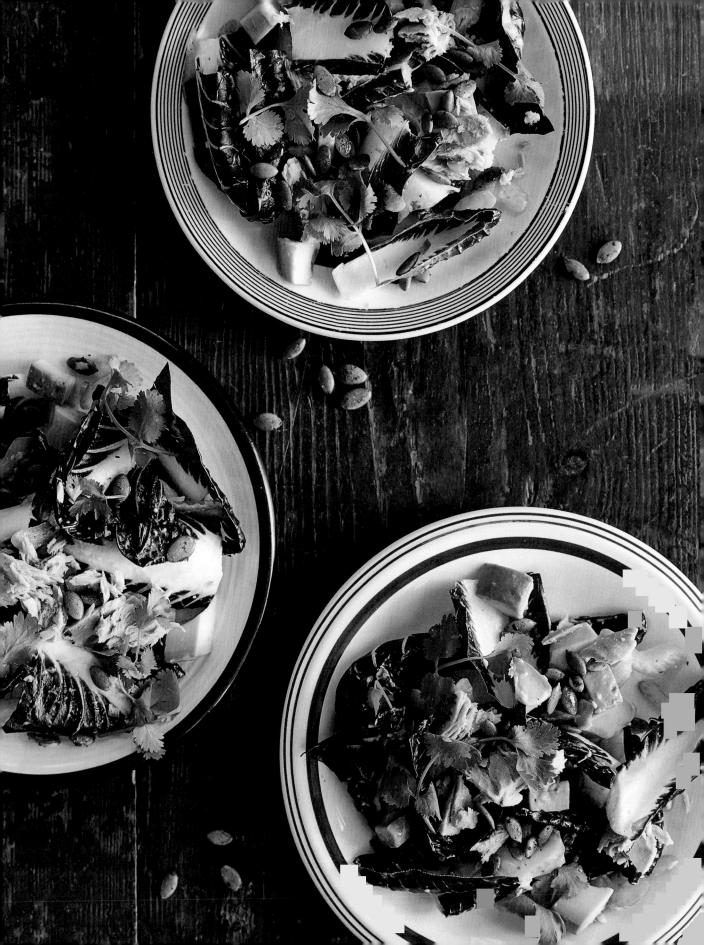

You use a whole avocado here, half for the salad and half for the dressing. In the salad, its richness offsets the bitterness of the radicchio and the heat of the chile. In the dressing, it balances the tartness of tomatillos. Altogether, that single avocado makes this tuna salad satisfying enough to be a light lunch.

SERVES
4 TO 6

CELERY AND TREVISO RADICCHIO SALAD WITH SPICED PEPITAS

5 large celery stalks, very thinly sliced

2 heads Treviso radicchio, torn into large pieces

½ avocado, peeled and cut into ½-inch dice

I Anaheim chile, stemmed, seeded, and very thinly sliced

Avocado-Tomatillo Vinaigrette (recipe follows)

2 ounces high-quality tuna packed in olive oil, preferably ventresca (see page 46), flaked

Spiced Pepitas (page 303)

Cilantro leaves

In a large bowl, toss the celery, radicchio, avocado, and chile until evenly mixed, then drizzle in the vinaigrette. Gently toss until well coated.

Top with the tuna, pepitas, and cilantro and serve immediately.

RECIPE CONTINUES ▶

AVOCADO-TOMATILLO VINAIGRETTE MAKES ABOUT ⅔ CUP

Like a cross between guacamole and salsa verde, this dressing would be delicious with any Mexican-inspired salad. You could also shave crunchy vegetables, such as kohlrabi, to eat as "chips" with this "dip."

2 tomatillos, husked

½ avocado, peeled and diced

½ garlic clove, grated on a Microplane

Juice of ½ lime

2 tablespoons fresh cilantro

2 tablespoons white balsamic vinegar

Coarse sea salt

½ cup extra-virgin olive oil

1 In a cast-iron skillet, cook the tomatillos over high heat, turning occasionally, until evenly charred, 12 to 14 minutes. Transfer to a blender and cool.

2 When the tomatillos are cool, add the avocado, garlic, lime juice, cilantro, vinegar, and a generous pinch of salt. Blend until smooth. With the machine running, add the olive oil. Season with salt.

VENTRESCA TUNA

When I first started cooking professionally in Spain, I fell in love with the country's incredible high-quality jarred tuna packed in olive oil. This protein powerhouse is now a staple in my home and restaurants. Of all the great types of Spanish tuna available, none is better than *ventresca*, which is cut from the belly. (In raw form at sushi bars, it's known as *toro*.) It's deeply flavorful and almost buttery in its rich, silken texture. Keep some on hand to instantly elevate meals by popping open a jar.

When summer produce is at its best, I don't bother cooking it at all. I pull out my mandoline to cut everything into paper-thin slices so that each bite combines freshness with crunch (see page 36). This is the perfect dinner for a hot day. It also holds up in lunch boxes, so you don't have to settle for fast-food crap.

SERVES
4 TO 6

SUMMER SQUASH SALAD WITH RADISHES AND TUNA

12 ounces mixed summer squash, such as small zucchini, yellow squash, and pattypans, cut into paper-thin rounds

4 ounces mixed radishes, such as red, watermelon, and cello, cut into paper-thin rounds

4 ounces best-quality tuna packed in olive oil, flaked into large chunks

2 shallots, cut into paper-thin rings

24 Sun Gold tomatoes, halved

1 serrano chile, thinly sliced

1 cup paper-thin slices raw purple cauliflower

¾ cup extra-virgin olive oil

Juice of 4 limes, rinds reserved

Jacobsen flake finishing sea salt and freshly ground black pepper

Chopped fresh dill and cilantro, for serving

1 (1-ounce) chunk Parmesan cheese

In a large bowl, toss the squash, radishes, tuna, shallots, tomatoes, chile, cauliflower, olive oil, and lime juice. Season with salt and pepper.

Divide among serving plates and top with the fresh herbs. Zest the lime rinds directly on top, then use a vegetable peeler to shave the Parmesan on top. Serve immediately.

Mixing temperatures and textures makes this early spring salad both warming and refreshing. Some of the cauliflower and artichokes get sautéed in chunks, along with white asparagus, and the rest are shaved raw, along with celery root. A honey-Dijon vinaigrette brings everything together, whisked with the added depth of the oil used to cook the vegetables.

CAULIFLOWER, CELERIAC, WHITE ASPARAGUS, AND ARTICHOKE SALAD

I head cauliflower, halved and cored

4 tablespoons grass-fed unsalted butter

½ teaspoon ground coriander

Coarse sea salt and freshly ground black pepper

2 lemons

¼ cup extra-virgin olive oil, preferably Arbequina

2 artichokes, prepped (see page 38)

8 stalks white asparagus, trimmed, peeled, and cut into 2-inch batons

I small celery root, trimmed and peeled

I cup chopped frisée

2 tablespoons champagne vinegar

I garlic clove, grated on a Microplane

I teaspoon honey

I teaspoon Dijon mustard

Fresh basil leaves

Cut half the cauliflower into paper-thin slices with a mandoline. Cut the remaining florets into 1-inch pieces.

In a large skillet, melt the butter over medium-high heat until it begins to get foamy and starts to turn brownish and give off a lovely, nutty aroma, about 4 minutes. Add the cauliflower florets and cook, stirring often, until golden, 3 to 5 minutes. Drain on paper towels and sprinkle with the coriander and a pinch each of salt and pepper. Zest 1 lemon on top and let cool completely.

Wipe out the skillet with a paper towel and add the olive oil. Set over low heat.

Cut one artichoke into ½-inch pieces and put it in the hot oil, along with the white asparagus. Cook, stirring occasionally, until just tender, about 6 minutes. Remove from the heat and let cool in the oil.

While the vegetables cool, cut the celery root and remaining artichoke into paper-thin slices on the mandoline. Transfer to a large bowl and add the cauliflower slices and florets and frisée. Transfer the sautéed asparagus and artichoke to the bowl, leaving the cooking oil in the pan. Season with salt and pepper and toss gently.

In a small bowl, whisk together the vinegar, garlic, honey, and mustard. While whisking, add the reserved cooking oil in a slow, steady stream. Whisk until emulsified.

Zest the remaining lemon on top of the vegetables and squeeze in the juice of both lemons. Drizzle the vinaigrette over, then toss again until everything is evenly coated.

Transfer to serving plates. Tear basil leaves and scatter them on top. Serve immediately.

WHITE ASPARAGUS

Fresh spears are available at specialty markets in early spring. They're expensive because they're tough to grow, but they're worth it. They're sweeter and more tender than green asparagus, but still have lots of vitamins C and A.

Think of this as a lettuce cup or composed crudités. The gondola-shaped radicchio leaves cradle tomatoes and parsley doused with a savory tuna dressing, and taste best when eaten by hand. You can also turn it into a fork-and-knife meal by topping it with toasted walnuts, boiled eggs, and shaved Parmesan.

SERVES
2 TO 4

TREVISO RADICCHIO AND PARSLEY SALAD WITH TONNATO DRESSING

2 heads Treviso radicchio, leaves separated	½ cup grape or cherry tomatoes, halved	¼ cup fresh flat-leaf parsley leaves Tonnato Dressing (recipe follows)

Arrange the radicchio leaves on a serving platter, cupped-side up. Scatter the tomatoes and parsley on top, then drizzle the dressing in the cups. Eat with your hands!

TONNATO DRESSING MAKES ABOUT ⅔ CUP

Tonnato is a classic Italian sauce from the Piedmont region made by blending tuna until creamy. It's traditionally slathered all over veal for the dish *vitello tonnato*, but I like the flavor with vegetables. My lightened version, with a hint of sweetness from white balsamic vinegar, can be drizzled onto salads or used as a dip for crudités.

¼ cup high-quality tuna packed in olive oil	¼ cup white balsamic vinegar
1 tablespoon whole-grain Dijon mustard	¼ cup extra-virgin olive oil
1 teaspoon grated peeled fresh horseradish	Jacobsen flake finishing sea salt and freshly ground black pepper
¼ garlic clove, grated on a Microplane	

In a blender, combine the tuna, mustard, horseradish, garlic, and vinegar and puree until smooth. With the machine running, add the olive oil and blend until emulsified. Season with salt and pepper.

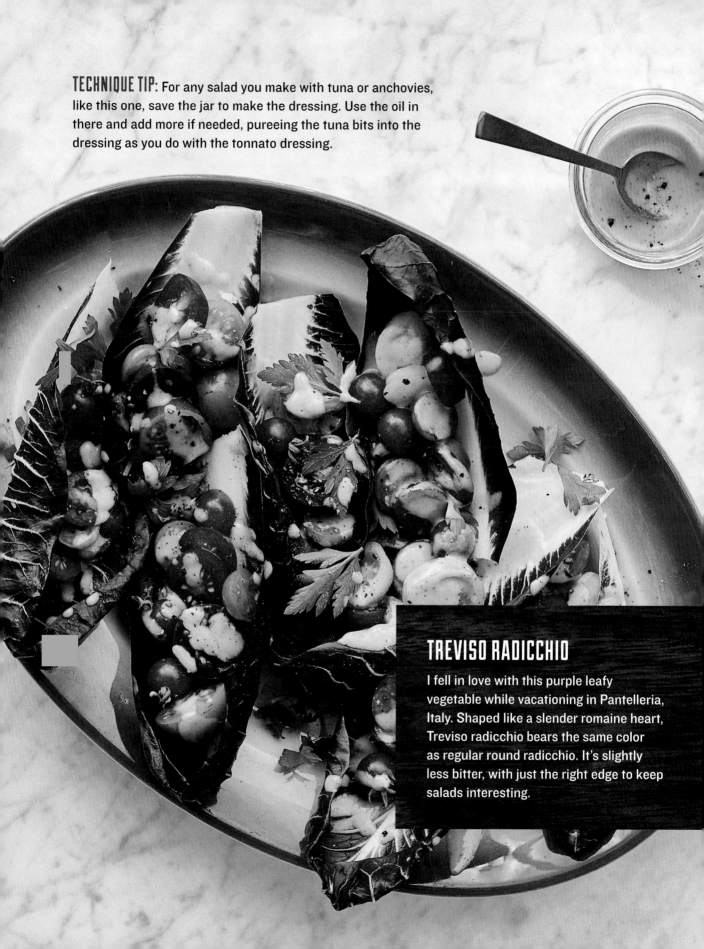

TECHNIQUE TIP: For any salad you make with tuna or anchovies, like this one, save the jar to make the dressing. Use the oil in there and add more if needed, pureeing the tuna bits into the dressing as you do with the tonnato dressing.

TREVISO RADICCHIO

I fell in love with this purple leafy vegetable while vacationing in Pantelleria, Italy. Shaped like a slender romaine heart, Treviso radicchio bears the same color as regular round radicchio. It's slightly less bitter, with just the right edge to keep salads interesting.

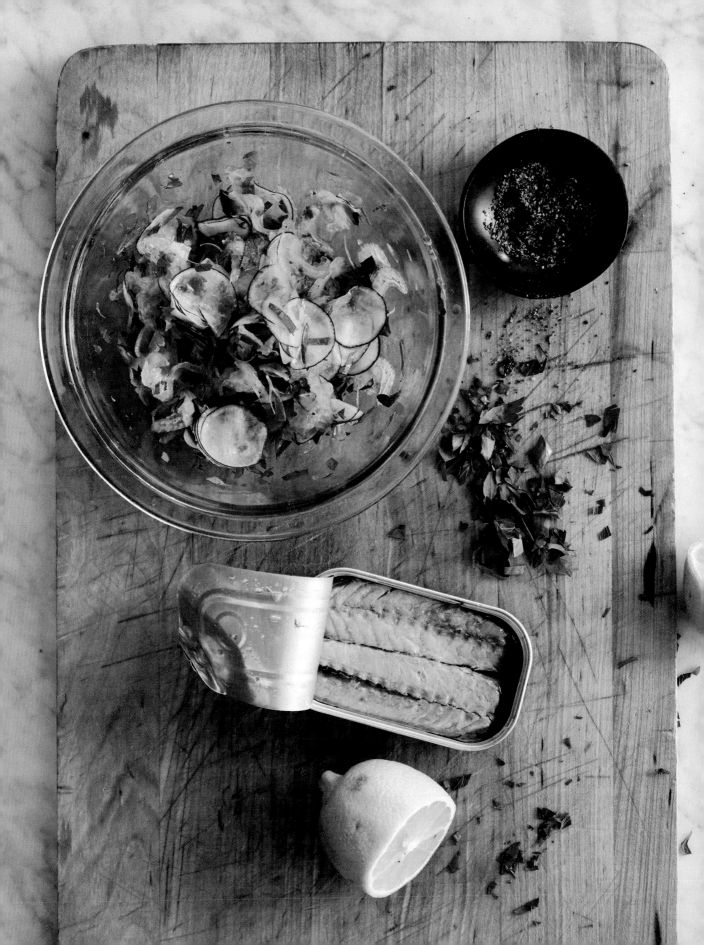

When I need a quick, tasty, and nutritious lunch, I'll make myself this salad. It takes a minute and a half to throw together. It's not what most people think of when they think of salad. It's more like what you'd get when you order antipasti at a restaurant in Italy. I figured, "Why not have their snack as my meal?" It's easy and made with ingredients available year-round. There's not much to it, but it's so delicious.

SERVES 1

CELERY AND RADISH SALAD WITH MACKEREL

I celery stalk, very thinly sliced

3 red radishes, thinly sliced

1½ tablespoons extra-virgin olive oil

Juice of I lemon

2 tablespoons chopped fresh flat-leaf parsley

Jacobsen flake finishing sea salt and freshly ground black pepper

I (4.4-ounce) can wild mackerel packed in olive oil

Espelette pepper

In a large bowl, toss the celery, radishes, olive oil, lemon juice, and parsley with salt and black pepper until well mixed. Flake the fish into the mix and top with a pinch of Espelette.

CANNED WILD MACKEREL IN OLIVE OIL

Stash them in your pantry. They're an instant—and delicious—source of omega-3 fatty acids. You can throw them onto any salad or simply cooked greens. I like Cole's brand, but try what you can find and stock up on your favorite.

Pesto may be associated with pasta, but it's amazing in salads, too. You can swap in any pesto here, but I really love the bite of the garlic scapes with peppery arugula and salty prosciutto and Parm.

SERVES
2 TO 4

ARUGULA AND CUCUMBER SALAD WITH PROSCIUTTO AND PARMESAN

2 tablespoons Garlic Scape and Pistachio Pesto (page 293)

¼ cup extra-virgin olive oil

2 tablespoons sherry vinegar

5 ounces baby arugula

½ seedless cucumber, thinly sliced

Jacobsen flake finishing sea salt and freshly ground black pepper

I ounce sliced prosciutto

I ounce Parmesan cheese, shaved

1 In a large bowl, whisk together the pesto, olive oil, and vinegar. Add the arugula and cucumber and lightly season with salt and pepper. Gently toss until evenly coated.

2 Divide among serving plates and top with the prosciutto and Parmesan. Serve immediately.

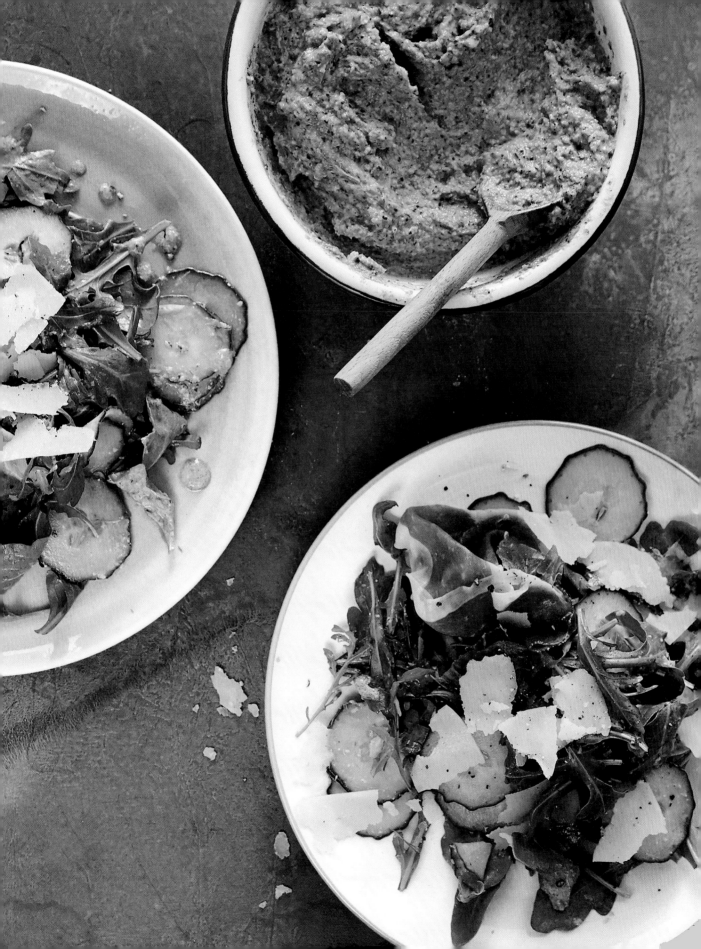

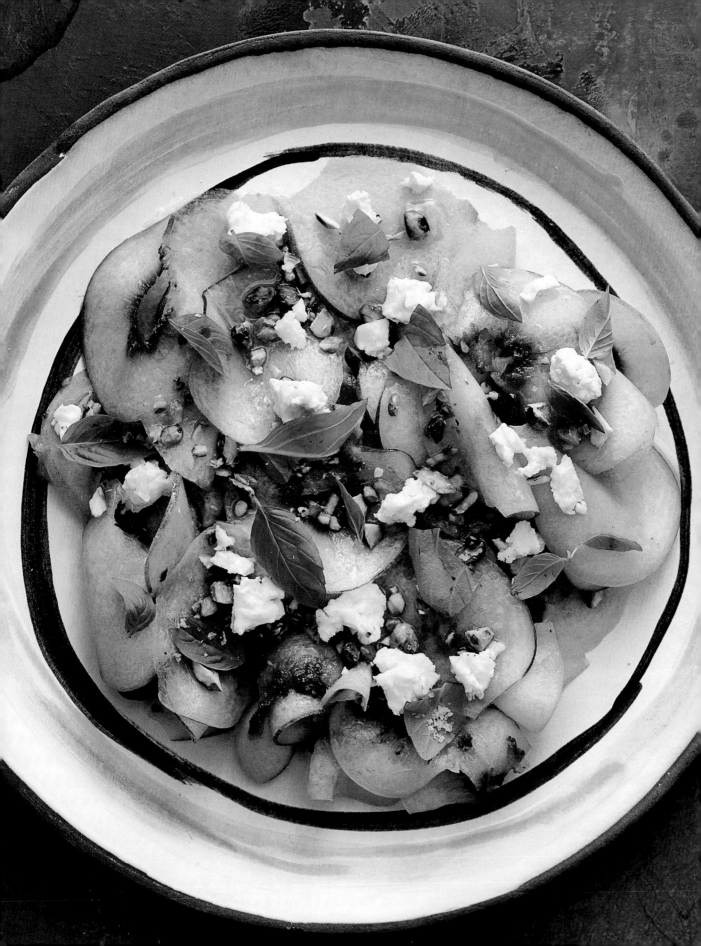

I often find that simplest is best. One day, while I was eating a classic summer tomato Caprese salad, I thought, "Why can't you treat other fruit in the same way?" This is totally a tomato salad, but with peaches. It's the sort of thing I make for lunch during bike tours I lead.

SLICED PEACHES WITH FETA, PISTACHIOS, AND HONEY

1 tablespoon shelled unsalted pistachios

2 slightly underripe yellow peaches, halved, pitted, and cut into ⅛-inch-thick slices

2 tablespoons crumbled sheep's-milk feta cheese

Jacobsen flake finishing sea salt and freshly ground black pepper

Extra-virgin olive oil

Raw honey

Fresh basil leaves

In a small skillet, cook the pistachios over high heat, tossing often, until browned in spots, about 3 minutes. Let cool completely, then chop.

Arrange the peaches on a serving plate and top with the nuts and cheese. Sprinkle with salt and pepper and drizzle with olive oil and honey. Tear the basil leaves and scatter them over the top. Serve immediately.

PAIRING TIP: **Basil + Fruit:** I love basil with fruit. When I was in my late teens, I was really into baking bread. I had been playing around with an apple-based sourdough starter, so I decided to put apples in the dough. I went out to the garden, plucked some basil, and threw it in, too. That loaf was so delicious. The aroma from the basil was a revelation. I've been loving the marriage of basil and fruit since—but now without any grains.

Both arugula and walnuts have faint bitter notes that go so well with sweet stone fruit. You can swap in peaches for the nectarines here. In either case, be sure to keep the basil, which highlights their honeyed flavor.

ARUGULA AND NECTARINE SALAD WITH WALNUTS

2 cups baby arugula

2 nectarines, pitted and cut into chunks

⅓ cup walnuts, toasted

12 fresh basil leaves, torn

Cider Honey Vinaigrette (recipe follows)

Jacobsen flake finishing sea salt and freshly ground black pepper

⅓ cup crumbled sheep's-milk feta cheese

1   In a large bowl, combine the arugula, nectarines, walnuts, and basil. Drizzle on the vinaigrette and gently toss with your hands until everything is well coated.

2   Transfer to serving plates and season with salt and pepper. Scatter the cheese on top and serve immediately.

CIDER HONEY VINAIGRETTE MAKES ABOUT ⅔ CUP

This is the ideal dressing for any salad that combines greens, especially bitter ones, with fruit.

¼ cup raw apple cider vinegar

2 teaspoons whole-grain Dijon mustard

2 teaspoons raw honey

½ garlic clove, grated on a Microplane

½ cup extra-virgin olive oil

Pinch of coarse sea salt

Combine all the ingredients in a jar, cover tightly, and shake well. Rock and roll until it's pretty emulsified.

Is this a salad? A dessert? A savory dish? You tell me. I like the idea of flirting with eating conventions. There are so many interplays between sweet and savory and sour here: the big flakes of salt on the succulent fruit, the tanginess of the vinaigrette and lime juice. And all of it is so good for you. You can have it for breakfast, lunch, dinner, snack, or dessert and it'll feel right.

SERVES
2 TO 4

SLICED PAPAYA WITH TURMERIC-CHIA VINAIGRETTE AND KEY LIMES

I ripe papaya

Jacobsen flake finishing sea salt

Turmeric–Chia Seed Vinaigrette (recipe follows)

6 key limes, halved

Cilantro leaves

Cut the papaya in half and scoop out and discard the seeds. Cut each half into eighths lengthwise, then cut off the peel. Cut each eighth crosswise into 1-inch pieces.

Arrange the papaya on serving plates and sprinkle with salt. Spoon the vinaigrette on top, then arrange the lime halves on top for squeezing. Garnish with cilantro and serve immediately.

KEY LIMES

What we call key limes are regular limes in other parts of the world. They're so frigging good! Instead of being straight-up sour, they have a floral, fruity brightness.

RECIPE CONTINUES ▶

TURMERIC–CHIA SEED VINAIGRETTE MAKES ABOUT ½ CUP

Turmeric is a fantastic anti-inflammatory and adds a welcome bitter note to this dressing, which is especially good on fruit.

I teaspoon chia seeds

3 tablespoons citrus champagne vinegar

5 tablespoons extra-virgin olive oil

I (2-inch) piece fresh turmeric, scrubbed

Combine the chia seeds, vinegar, and olive oil in a jar. Use a Microplane to grate the turmeric directly into the mixture. Cover, shake well, and let sit for at least 20 minutes for the chia seeds to bloom.

PAPAYA

This tropical fruit tastes like strawberry with a ripe fecundity. A good one turns to cream in your mouth, and that's what makes it so delicious. I can't deny the sensuality of this fruit. Split it open lengthwise and tell me you don't see what I see. In Venezuela, it's called *la lechosa*, which also means "milky" in a sexy way. That basically describes how it feels when you eat it, too.

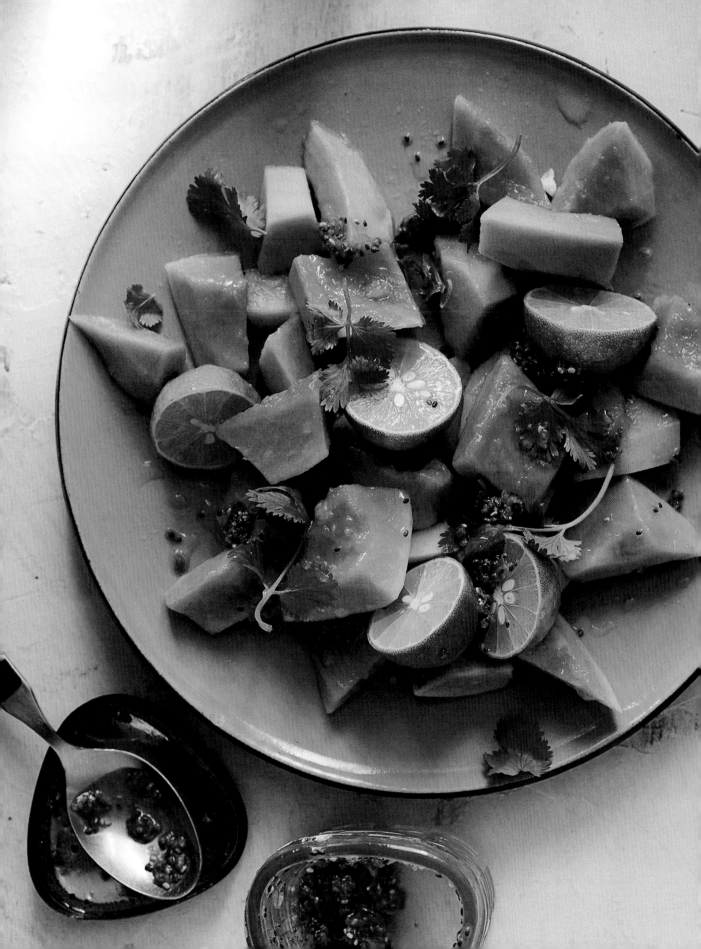

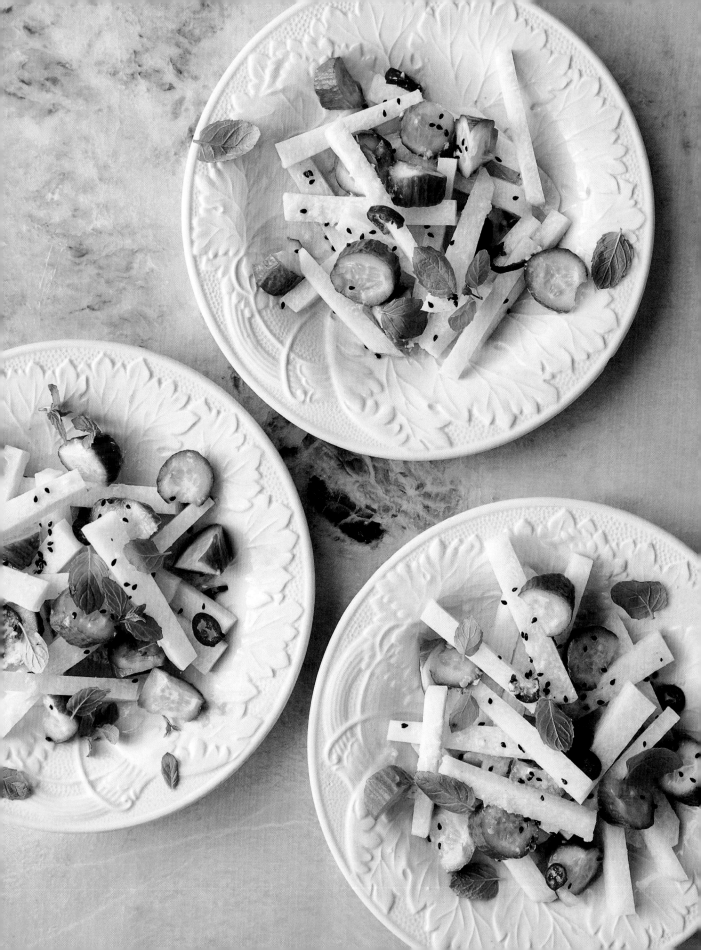

This dish has a slightly pickled taste. The flavor is more acidic than that of a typical salad, but not so sour that you can't eat a lot of it. If anything, the tart crunch of the jicama and cucumbers with the pop of sesame seeds is addictive. Serve this with Steamed Pistou-Rubbed Monkfish Fillets Wrapped in Collards (page 195) and you have an amazing meal.

SERVES
2 TO 4

CUCUMBER-JICAMA SALAD WITH CHILES

I small jicama, peeled, quartered, and cut into ¼-inch-thick sticks

2 mini cucumbers, cut into ½-inch-thick slices

½ Fresno chile, seeded, if desired, and very thinly sliced

Ginger Vinaigrette (recipe follows)

⅓ cup fresh mint leaves

I tablespoon black sesame seeds

Jacobsen flake finishing sea salt

1   In a large bowl, combine the jicama, cucumbers, and chile. Shake the vinaigrette well and pour it all over. Sprinkle mint leaves and sesame seeds over the top.

2   Gently toss with your hands until everything is well mixed. Season with salt. Serve immediately.

GINGER VINAIGRETTE MAKES ABOUT ½ CUP

This isn't so much a dressing as it is a way to season and draw out the flavor of wet vegetables like cucumbers by sucking the moisture out. You can use it with any chunky vegetable. It tastes best with the O brand of yuzu rice vinegar.

¼ cup rice vinegar, preferably yuzu rice vinegar

I (2-inch) piece fresh ginger, peeled

¼ cup extra-virgin olive oil

Put the vinegar in a jar and use a Microplane to grate the ginger directly into the vinegar. Add the olive oil, cover tightly, and shake well.

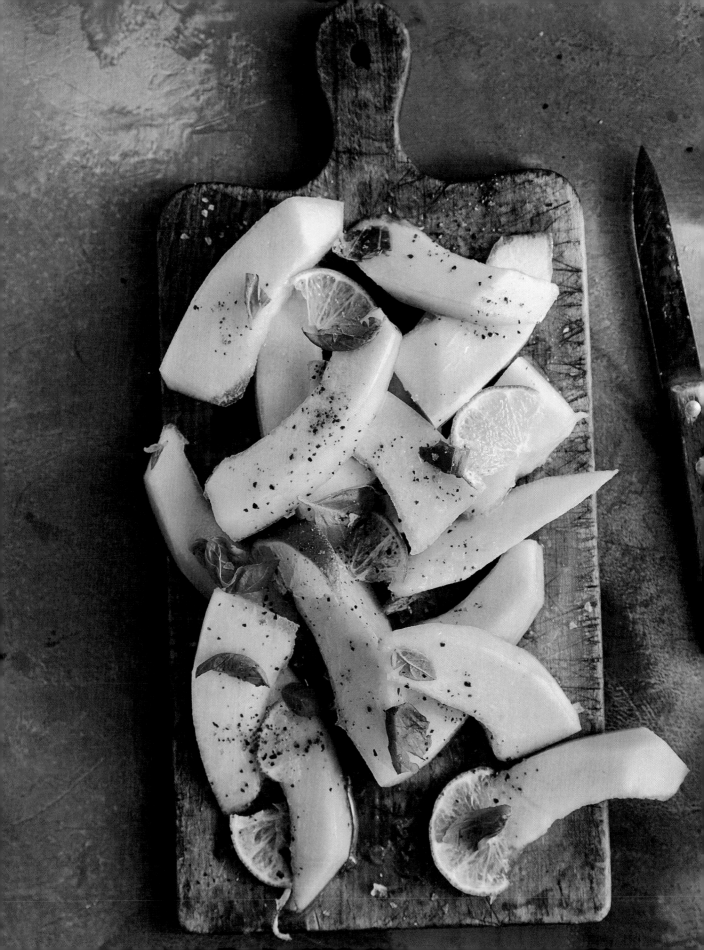

When I was eighteen, my grandmother Mutti and I traveled to Nicaragua for a community service trip. We stayed in this crappy hostel that had a chest freezer in the middle of the room filled with frozen melon. You could eat it straight up or ask them to puree it into juice. It was so refreshing. To this day, melon is something I love ice-cold. It's awesome on its own, but I like it even more when it's brightened with salt, chile, and lime.

HONEYDEW WITH OLIVE OIL, SEA SALT, ESPELETTE PEPPER, AND LIME

½ honeydew, peeled, seeded, cut into wedges, and chilled until very cold

Extra-virgin olive oil

Jacobsen flake finishing sea salt

Espelette pepper

Fresh basil leaves

½ lime, plus slices for serving

Scatter the honeydew in a single layer on a serving platter. Drizzle with olive oil and sprinkle with salt and Espelette. Tear the basil and scatter it on top. Squeeze the lime juice all over and serve immediately with lime slices.

JACOBSEN SALT CO. FLAKE FINISHING SEA SALT

You'll notice that I always call for this incredible stuff in my recipes. (Of course, you can always swap in another high-quality, flaked sea salt if you can't find Jacobsen.) As with any other ingredient, I always look for the best quality product from producers I respect. I first discovered this salt a few years ago and I've come to love it. Ben Jacobsen started harvesting and processing sea salt from the cold waters off the Oregon coast in 2011, and his company has grown to become a nationally recognized producer of some of the finest salts in the world. For a while, we demonized salt (not unlike the way in which we demonized fats) without recognizing that salt is essential to our bodies. Without it, we can't survive. While I don't advocate overconsumption of salt, I truly believe that refined sugar is the real problem when it comes to overconsumption.

Toasted pecans and garlic chives bring a surprising savory element to a classic summer salad. The good fats from the nuts make this really satisfying, too.

HEIRLOOM TOMATO AND WATERMELON SALAD WITH BURRATA

4 mixed heirloom tomatoes, cored and cut into 1-inch chunks (8 cups)

¼ watermelon, rind discarded, cut into 1-inch chunks (4 cups)

½ cup pecans, toasted

¼ cup minced garlic chives

¼ cup fresh basil leaves, torn

¼ cup fresh mint leaves, torn

Jacobsen flake finishing sea salt and freshly ground black pepper

Meyer Lemon Vinaigrette (recipe follows)

4 ounces burrata cheese

Extra-virgin olive oil

1   In a large bowl, combine the tomatoes, watermelon, pecans, chives, basil, and mint. Season with salt and pepper and gently toss to mix. Drizzle the vinaigrette all over and toss until everything is evenly coated.

2   Transfer to a serving platter. Tear the burrata into small chunks and scatter them on top. Drizzle with olive oil and sprinkle with salt. Serve immediately.

RECIPE CONTINUES ▶

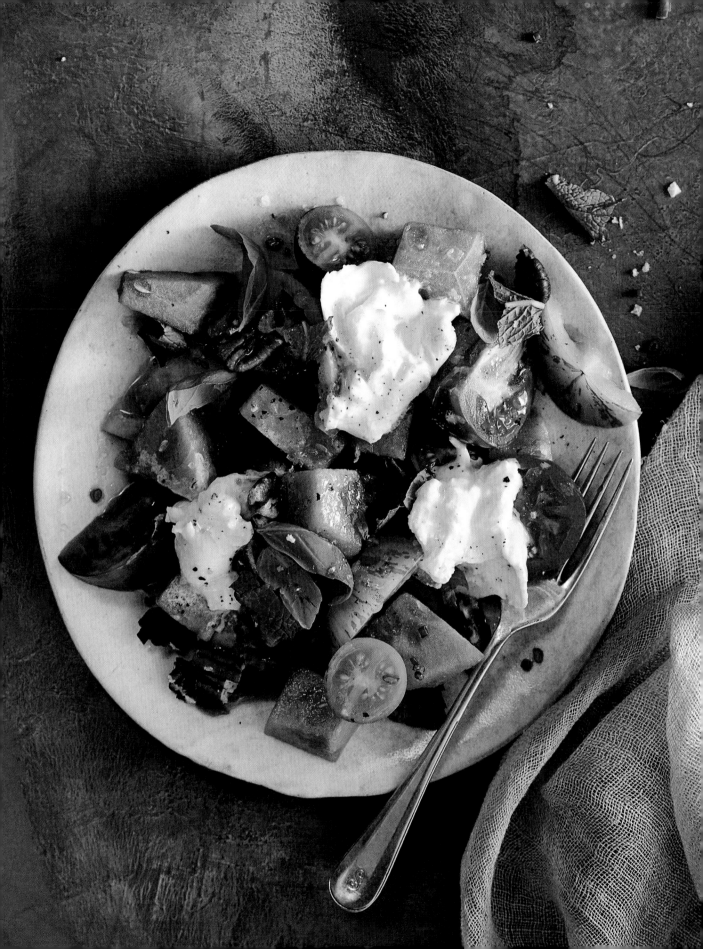

MEYER LEMON VINAIGRETTE MAKES ABOUT I CUP

Blending lemon zest into this dressing gives it body so it makes watery vegetables taste rich.

Zest and juice of I Meyer lemon

3 tablespoons champagne vinegar

I tablespoon raw honey

I tablespoon Dijon mustard

¼ garlic clove, grated on a Microplane

Coarse sea salt and freshly ground black pepper

¾ cup extra-virgin olive oil, preferably Arbequina

In a blender, combine the lemon zest, lemon juice, vinegar, honey, mustard, garlic, and a pinch each of salt and pepper. Puree until smooth. With the machine running, add the olive oil in a slow, steady stream. Puree until emulsified. Season with salt and pepper.

MEYER LEMONS

Meyer lemons, which have an almost sweet floral tartness, are now readily available in markets. Their measured sourness makes them ideal for dressings for acidic fruits and vegetables, like tomatoes.

Eating whole mushrooms raw is a little intense, but shave them carpaccio-style and they're so, so good. Creminis smell and taste like the forest to me, so I serve them with other forest-y flavors—pine nuts, thyme, and truffle. I finish the combination with Idiazábal cheese, a hard cow's-milk variety from Spain, for its nutty notes. If you can't find Idiazábal, Gruyère tastes great, too.

SERVES
1 TO 2

CREMINI CARPACCIO

1 ounce cremini mushrooms	1 tablespoon buttered pine nuts (recipe follows)	1 black truffle (optional)
1 lemon	2 tablespoons Brown Butter and Pine Nut Vinaigrette (recipe follows)	½ ounce Idiazábal cheese
Fleur de sel		½ teaspoon fresh thyme leaves, preferably lemon thyme
Espelette pepper		

1   Slice the cremini mushrooms as thinly as possible on a mandoline and arrange on a serving plate. Zest the lemon directly on top, then squeeze the juice from half the lemon all over. Sprinkle with fleur de sel and Espelette. Scatter the pine nuts on top.

2   Drizzle the vinaigrette all over. If you have a black truffle, grate a light dusting on top with a Microplane. Use the Microplane to grate the cheese over all. Sprinkle with the thyme leaves and serve immediately.

CREMINI MUSHROOMS

More mature than white buttons and younger than portobellos, these coffee-colored mushrooms, sometimes labeled baby bellas, have an earthy flavor. Studies have shown that they support the immune system and can regulate inflammation.

RECIPE CONTINUES ▶

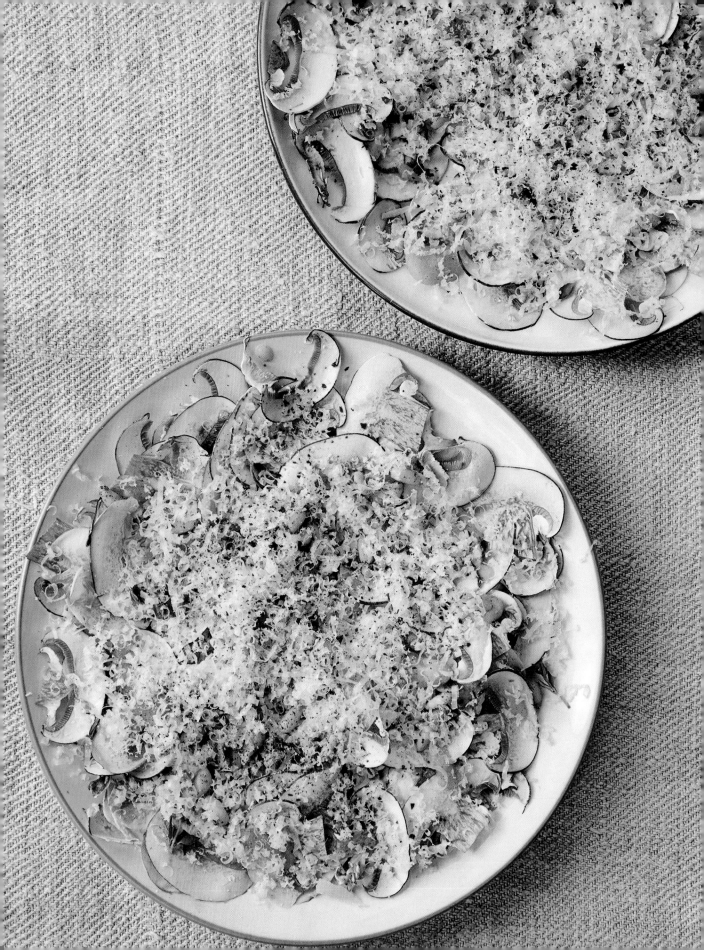

BROWN BUTTER AND PINE NUT VINAIGRETTE MAKES ABOUT ⅔ CUP

Good, grass-fed butter can—and should—be enjoyed. I like to brown it to bring out its nuttiness, then add nuts, too. Vinegar and lemon juice balance the richness, making this dressing especially good for mushrooms and root vegetables.

8 tablespoons grass-fed unsalted butter

I tablespoon pine nuts

I garlic clove, grated on a Microplane

2 tablespoons raw honey

¼ cup Moscatel or white balsamic vinegar

Juice of I lemon

Jacobsen flake finishing sea salt and freshly ground black pepper

Put the butter in a small skillet and set it over medium heat. Cook, stirring and scraping the pan often, until the milk solids separate and the butter smells and looks nutty brown. Skim off and discard any foamy milk solids that have risen to the top.

Reduce the heat to low. Add the pine nuts and gently toast the nuts to infuse the butter with their flavor. Once the nuts are light golden, strain the butter through a fine-mesh sieve into a small bowl. Reserve the nuts for the Cremini Carpaccio. Add the garlic and whisk well.

In a medium bowl, whisk together the honey, vinegar, and lemon juice. While whisking, add the butter mixture in a steady stream and whisk until emulsified. Season with salt and pepper.

Crunchy apple and kohlrabi fanned under torn olives and basil feels light and bright in the fall and winter when it's hard to get vibrant food on the table. To make this a heartier salad, crumble some goat cheese or feta on top. Or serve it as is with other fall salads or with a stew or braise.

APPLE AND SHAVED KOHLRABI WITH CASTELVETRANO OLIVES AND BASIL

1 tart crunchy apple, cored and cut into paper-thin slices on a mandoline

1 kohlrabi, cut into paper-thin slices on a mandoline

2 tablespoons raw apple cider vinegar

¼ cup extra-virgin olive oil

Jacobsen flake finishing sea salt

7 Castelvetrano olives, pitted and torn

Fresh basil leaves

In a large bowl, combine the apple, kohlrabi, vinegar, olive oil, and a big pinch of salt. Toss gently until everything is evenly coated. Transfer to a serving plate and top with the olives. Scatter the basil on top. Serve immediately.

CASTELVETRANO OLIVES

I love these olives because they're unpasteurized and not cured that long, which is why they're such a bright green color. That process keeps the taste and texture really fruity. Because the flesh clings hard to the pits, it's easier to pit and tear these olives by hand. That way, the pieces look nice and natural.

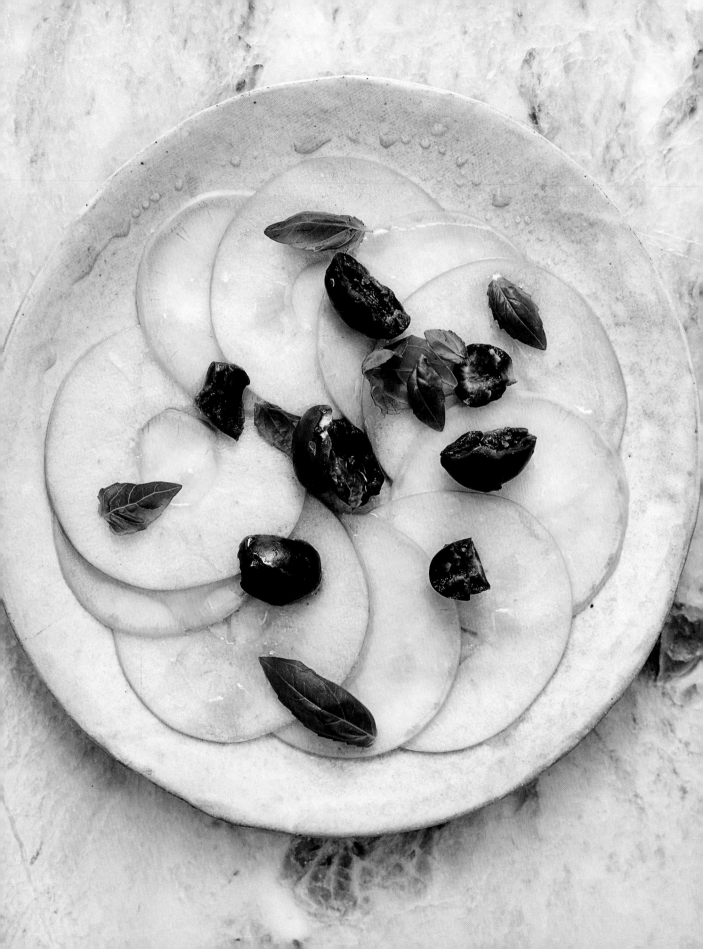

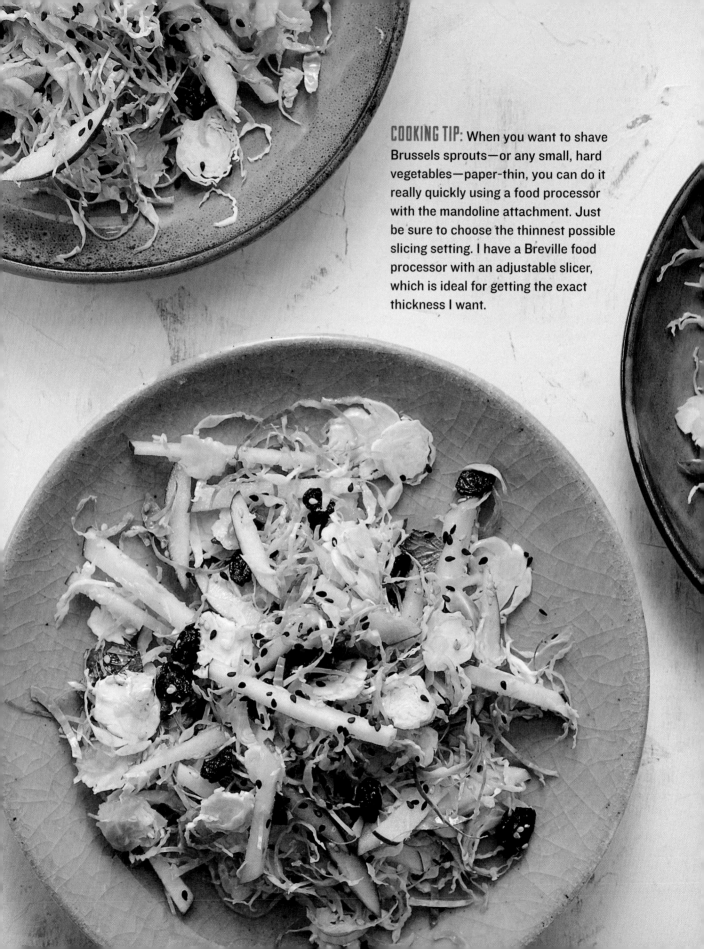

COOKING TIP: When you want to shave Brussels sprouts—or any small, hard vegetables—paper-thin, you can do it really quickly using a food processor with the mandoline attachment. Just be sure to choose the thinnest possible slicing setting. I have a Breville food processor with an adjustable slicer, which is ideal for getting the exact thickness I want.

My update on Asian slaw swaps Brussels sprouts for cabbage and apple for carrots. Using sesame in the dressing and salad doubles up on their good fats and makes this a good choice for anyone with nut allergies.

BRUSSELS SPROUTS AND DRIED CHERRY SALAD WITH BLACK AND WHITE SESAME

I pound Brussels sprouts, shaved paper-thin on a mandoline

I garlic clove, grated on a Microplane

I shallot, thinly sliced

I apple, cored and cut into matchsticks

I serrano chile, seeded and thinly sliced

¼ cup unsweetened dried tart cherries

Jacobsen flake finishing sea salt and freshly ground black pepper

Toasted Sesame Vinaigrette (recipe follows)

¼ cup chopped fresh mint

2 tablespoons black sesame seeds

In a large bowl, combine the Brussels sprouts, garlic, shallot, apple, chile, and dried cherries. Season with salt and pepper and toss well. Drizzle with the vinaigrette and toss until everything is evenly coated.

Transfer to serving dishes and scatter the mint and black sesame seeds all over.

TOASTED SESAME VINAIGRETTE MAKES ABOUT ¾ CUP

Like a rustic homemade tahini, this dressing tastes extra rich from a generous dose of sesame seeds. It pairs well with any Asian-inspired or Middle Eastern salad.

½ cup white sesame seeds, toasted

I garlic clove

Zest and juice of 2 lemons

I tablespoon raw honey

2 tablespoons white wine vinegar

¼ cup extra-virgin olive oil

Coarse sea salt and freshly ground black pepper

In a blender, puree the sesame seeds, garlic, lemon zest and juice, honey, and vinegar. With the machine running, add the oil in a stream. Season with salt and pepper.

One-bowl meals don't get better than this. You've got protein from the tuna, fiber and antioxidants from the quinoa and loads of vegetables, and just enough richness from nuts and goat cheese to keep you full until your next meal.

SERVES 4

QUINOA SALAD WITH CUCUMBERS, HERBS, AND TUNA

I lemon

Aromatic Tricolor Quinoa (page 307)

I seedless cucumber, scrubbed and cut into chunks

¼ cup pine nuts, toasted

2 cups baby arugula

I shallot, thinly sliced

I (6- to 7-ounce) can high-quality tuna packed in olive oil, drained and flaked

½ cup fresh mint, coarsely chopped

¼ cup fresh oregano leaves, coarsely chopped

Lemon Honey Mustard Vinaigrette (recipe follows)

Jacobsen flake finishing sea salt and freshly ground black pepper

½ cup crumbled goat cheese

1 Zest the lemon into a large bowl, then trim the top and bottom of the lemon. Use a paring knife to cut off all the pith and peel. Cut out the segments between the membranes and pick out any seeds. Cut the segments into small pieces and add to the bowl with the zest, along with the quinoa, cucumber, pine nuts, arugula, shallot, tuna, mint, and oregano.

2 Drizzle the vinaigrette on top and stir well until everything is evenly coated. Season with salt and pepper. Top with the goat cheese and serve.

RECIPE CONTINUES ▶

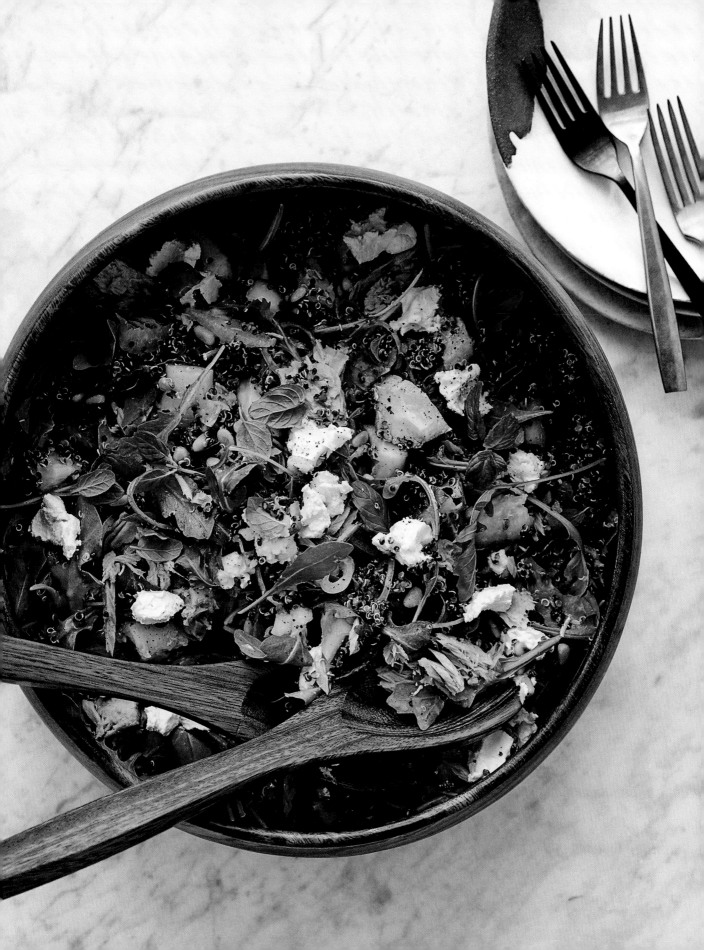

LEMON HONEY MUSTARD VINAIGRETTE MAKES ABOUT ⅓ CUP

Lemon lightens up the standard honey mustard combination, making it less cloying and more versatile. This is especially good with quinoa salads.

I garlic clove, grated on a Microplane

Zest of I lemon

2 tablespoons champagne vinegar

I teaspoon Dijon mustard

I teaspoon raw honey

¼ cup extra-virgin olive oil

Coarse sea salt and freshly ground black pepper

In a medium bowl, whisk together the garlic, lemon zest, vinegar, mustard, and honey until smooth. While whisking, add the olive oil in a slow, steady stream. Whisk until emulsified. Season with salt and pepper.

QUINOA

I stay away from grains, but quinoa isn't actually a grain, even though it cooks and eats like one. This pseudocereal is packed with antioxidants and healthy fats and is a great anti-inflammatory. When cooking it, be sure to start by rinsing the quinoa. You want to get rid of any remaining saponins that result in an unpleasant bitter taste.

Putting raw and roasted beets in a single salad shows off the range of these roots. Raw, they're snappy. Roasted, they're almost juicy. Arugula and horseradish offset their sweetness, while goat cheese brings all the textures together with creaminess.

SERVES
2 TO 4

MARINATED BEET SALAD WITH HORSERADISH VINAIGRETTE

I golden beet, peeled and cut into paper-thin slices on a mandoline

4 Roasted and Marinated Beets (page 264)

I cup sunflower sprouts

I cup arugula

½ cup hulled, unsalted sunflower seeds

Jacobsen flake finishing sea salt and freshly ground black pepper

Horseradish Vinaigrette (recipe follows)

I lemon

Fresh herbs, such as basil, mint, tarragon, dill, and thyme, torn

8 ounces goat cheese, preferably Humboldt Fog

Combine all the beets, the sprouts, arugula, and sunflower seeds in a large bowl. Season with salt and pepper and toss, then drizzle on the vinaigrette and toss until everything is evenly coated.

Transfer to a serving platter. Zest the lemon over the top, then scatter fresh herbs all over. Crumble the cheese on top and serve immediately.

RECIPE CONTINUES ▶

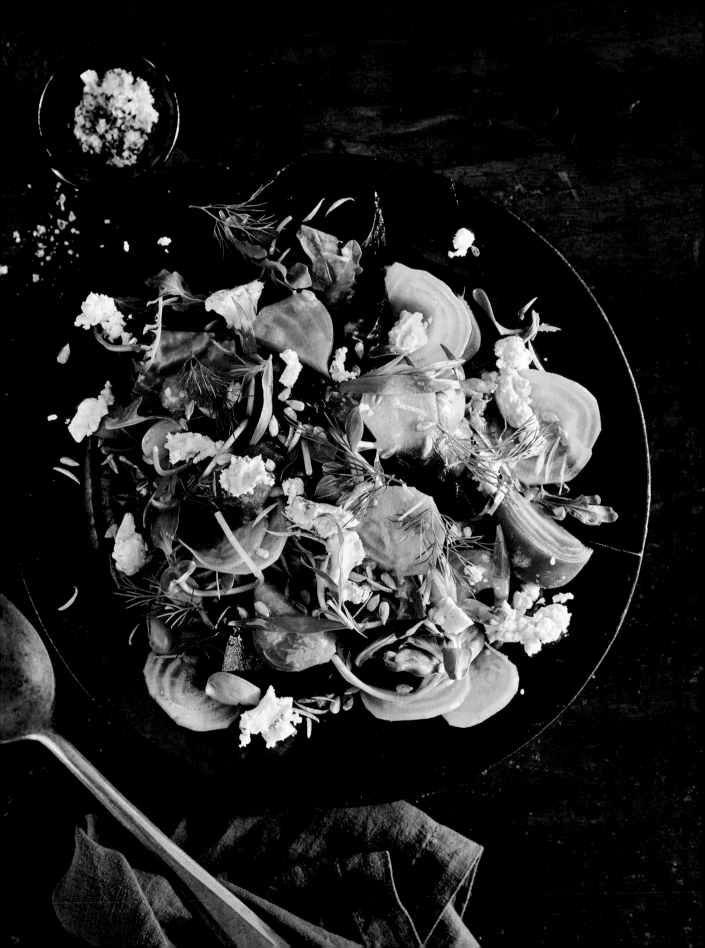

HORSERADISH VINAIGRETTE MAKES ABOUT ¾ CUP

Honey mellows sharp horseradish in this dressing-with-a-kick. It's especially good with sweet root vegetables and would also be nice with salmon.

3 tablespoons grated peeled fresh horseradish

I tablespoon Dijon mustard

I tablespoon raw honey

½ garlic clove, finely chopped

3 tablespoons white wine vinegar

6 tablespoons extra-virgin olive oil

Coarse sea salt and freshly ground black pepper

In a small bowl, whisk together the horseradish, mustard, honey, garlic, vinegar, and olive oil until well combined. Season with salt and pepper. Whisk again before using.

HORSERADISH

Fresh horseradish root shares the same bite as the jarred stuff, but tastes so much brighter. Plus, it's even better for you when fresh. Horseradish is in the same family as cruciferous vegetables and packs nutrients and minerals like folate and potassium. Simply grate it with a Microplane for its mustardy kick.

Squash rules this salad. Three varieties get roasted, blanched, and pickled, delivering a ton of different textures and flavors along with squash seeds. The resulting dish is as visually rewarding as it is delicious. All the colors of fall come together on one plate.

AUTUMN SQUASH SALAD

Kosher salt

1 delicata squash, halved, seeded, and thinly sliced

1 cup pickling liquid (see page 268)

¼ Hubbard squash, peeled, seeded, and cut into very thin ribbons on a mandoline

1 kabocha squash, cut into thin wedges and seeded

Jacobsen flake finishing sea salt and freshly ground black pepper

¼ cup extra-virgin olive oil, plus more for drizzling

¼ cup raw apple cider vinegar

1 teaspoon raw honey

1 garlic clove, grated on a Microplane

1 bunch Tuscan kale, stemmed, leaves torn into bite-size pieces

1 watermelon radish, greens chopped, radish cut into paper-thin slices on a mandoline

¼ cup pepitas (hulled pumpkin seeds), toasted

2 cups fresh cilantro leaves

½ ounce very thinly sliced jamón Serrano, prosciutto, or cured country ham

1   Bring a saucepan of generously salted water to a boil. Fill a large bowl with ice and salted water. Drop the delicata squash into the boiling water and cook until bright and crisp-tender, 2 to 3 minutes. Drain and immediately transfer to the ice water. When cool, drain again.

2   Preheat the oven to 375°F.

3   In a medium saucepan, heat the pickling liquid over medium-high heat. Add the Hubbard squash ribbons and simmer until tender, about 5 minutes. Set aside to cool in the liquid.

4   Put the kabocha squash wedges in a roasting pan, season with salt and pepper, and drizzle with olive oil. Toss until evenly coated and spread in a single layer. Roast until tender, about 25 minutes.

5   In a large bowl, whisk together the vinegar, honey, and garlic. While whisking, add the olive oil in a slow, steady stream. Continue whisking until emulsified. Add the kale, sliced radish and radish greens, pepitas, cilantro, and all three squashes. Toss until well coated. Season with salt and pepper.

6   Transfer to serving plates and lay the ham on top. Serve immediately.

RAW APPLE CIDER VINEGAR

Unfiltered, unpasteurized cider vinegar, with the "mother" of the vinegar floating around the cloudy liquid like a jellyfish, is an easy, great way to boost the good bacteria in your gut. Plus, it tastes less harsh than regular cider vinegar. Use it in dressings or toss any raw vegetables with it for a super-quick pickle.

When I eat out, I go for Japanese food. I love seaweed salad and carrot-ginger dressing on green salads, so I've combined them here. While some of the ingredients in this recipe aren't readily available at all supermarkets, most Asian and natural and organic food stores will carry a selection of Japanese ingredients. For the pantry items, order them online. I soak the seaweeds first according to the package directions because each variety differs slightly. I soak kombu in hot water, hijiki in cold. As a rule, I find the amounts generally double in volume after soaking. After soaking, I drain well and squeeze dry for fully prepared seaweed.

SERVES 2 TO 4

SEAWEED SALAD WITH CARROT-GINGER DRESSING

½ cup prepared dulse (see headnote)

½ cup thinly sliced prepared kombu (see headnote)

¼ cup prepared hijiki (see headnote)

2 nori sheets, crumbled

1 cup mustard greens, chopped

1 cup dandelion greens or mizuna

¼ cup daikon sprouts

½ daikon, sliced into paper-thin coins with a mandoline

1 king oyster mushroom, cut into paper-thin slices with a mandoline

Jacobsen flake finishing sea salt and freshly ground black pepper

Carrot-Ginger Vinaigrette (recipe follows)

4 shiso leaves, thinly sliced

2 tablespoons black sesame seeds

2 tablespoons white sesame seeds

1   In a large bowl, combine the dulse, kombu, hijiki, nori, mustard and dandelion greens, daikon sprouts and slices, and mushroom. Season with salt and pepper and toss gently. Drizzle with the vinaigrette and toss until everything is evenly coated.

2   Divide among serving dishes and top with the shiso and sesame seeds.

RECIPE CONTINUES ▶

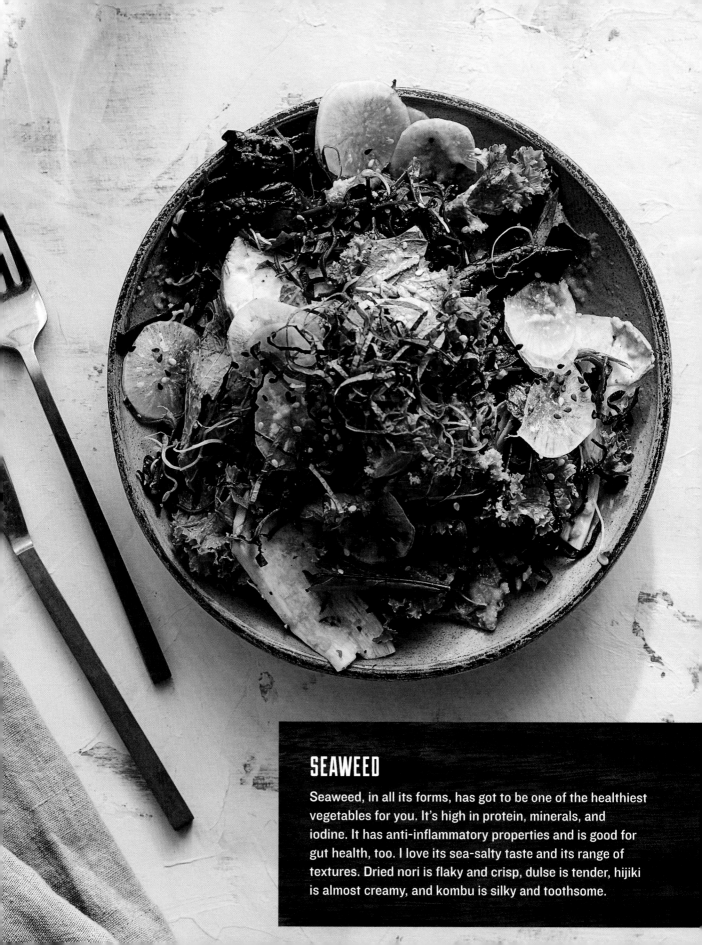

SEAWEED

Seaweed, in all its forms, has got to be one of the healthiest vegetables for you. It's high in protein, minerals, and iodine. It has anti-inflammatory properties and is good for gut health, too. I love its sea-salty taste and its range of textures. Dried nori is flaky and crisp, dulse is tender, hijiki is almost creamy, and kombu is silky and toothsome.

CARROT-GINGER VINAIGRETTE MAKES ABOUT ⅔ CUP

Kosher salt

I carrot

I tablespoon chopped peeled fresh ginger

I tablespoon shiro (white) miso

I garlic clove

2 tablespoons raw honey

⅓ cup rice vinegar

2 tablespoons Asian sesame oil

Coarse sea salt and freshly ground black pepper

Bring a small saucepan of generously salted water to a boil. Fill a medium bowl with ice and salted water. Add the carrot to the boiling water and cook until bright orange and crisp-tender, about 5 minutes. Transfer to the ice water. When cool, drain well, chop, and transfer to a blender.

Add the ginger, miso, garlic, honey, vinegar, and sesame oil to the blender and puree until smooth. Season with sea salt and pepper.

SHIRO (WHITE) MISO

Shiro miso, sometimes called white or blonde miso for its pale straw color, is a Japanese fermented soybean and rice paste. It's not only salty but filled with umami, that savory fifth taste that makes dishes irresistible and balances really nicely with acid in salad dressings. The fermentation process also makes miso a source of beneficial gut bacteria.

Root vegetables are often roasted to bring out their sweetness. Here I'm showing off their savory side, keeping them raw and coating them with a salty anchovy dressing. You can make this with any combination of roots, but the mix below is my favorite.

SHAVED ROOT VEGETABLE SALAD WITH BLOOD ORANGES

2 beets, preferably one candy-stripe and one gold

3 Jerusalem artichokes

7 English breakfast or red radishes

4 round red radishes

1 small watermelon radish

1 blood orange

3 tablespoons Anchovy-Citrus Vinaigrette (recipe follows), plus more to taste

Fresh dill and cilantro sprigs

Jacobsen flake finishing sea salt

1   Scrub all the vegetables under cold water until the grit is gone, then rub them dry. Using a mandoline, the slicer plate of a food processor, or a very sharp knife, cut all the vegetables into paper-thin slices. Transfer to a large bowl.

2   Zest the orange directly over the vegetables and toss until well mixed. Add the vinaigrette and toss until the vegetables are evenly coated. Taste and add more vinaigrette as desired. Divide among serving plates.

3   Peel the orange, separate the segments, and cut each into ½-inch pieces. Scatter over the salads, along with the dill and cilantro. Sprinkle with salt and serve.

RECIPE CONTINUES ▶

ANCHOVY-CITRUS VINAIGRETTE MAKES ABOUT 2 CUPS

Using a mortar and pestle to smash the anchovies releases their good oils and their flavor. Once all the other ingredients are stirred in, the anchovies are barely perceptible. They just bring a deep sea-salty richness.

2 anchovy fillets, with 1½ teaspoons oil
    from the container

4 strips lemon zest, peeled with a vegetable
    peeler

1 small garlic clove

Pinch of Espelette pepper or red pepper flakes

¼ cup plus 1 teaspoon white wine vinegar

1 tablespoon chopped fresh dill or cilantro

½ cup plus 1 tablespoon extra-virgin olive oil

1 teaspoon whole-grain Dijon mustard

Jacobsen flake finishing sea salt and freshly
    ground black pepper

In a mortar, combine the anchovies with their oil, lemon zest, garlic, Espelette, and 1 teaspoon of the vinegar. Gently smash with the pestle until the garlic cracks. Once it does, pound the mixture until the garlic and anchovies are pasty and the zest is finely broken. Add the dill and 1 tablespoon of the olive oil and smash with the pestle until the mixture is like paste. Scrape into a jar and add the mustard and remaining oil and vinegar. Cover tightly and shake well. Season with salt and pepper and shake again.

ANCHOVIES

Anchovies often get a bad rap, but that's because too many people associate their flavor with the overly fishy taste of cheap anchovies on pizza. Good anchovies are often packaged in glass jars with olive oil and have omega-3 fatty acids, an integral healthy fat that helps with the production of healthy HDL cholesterol.

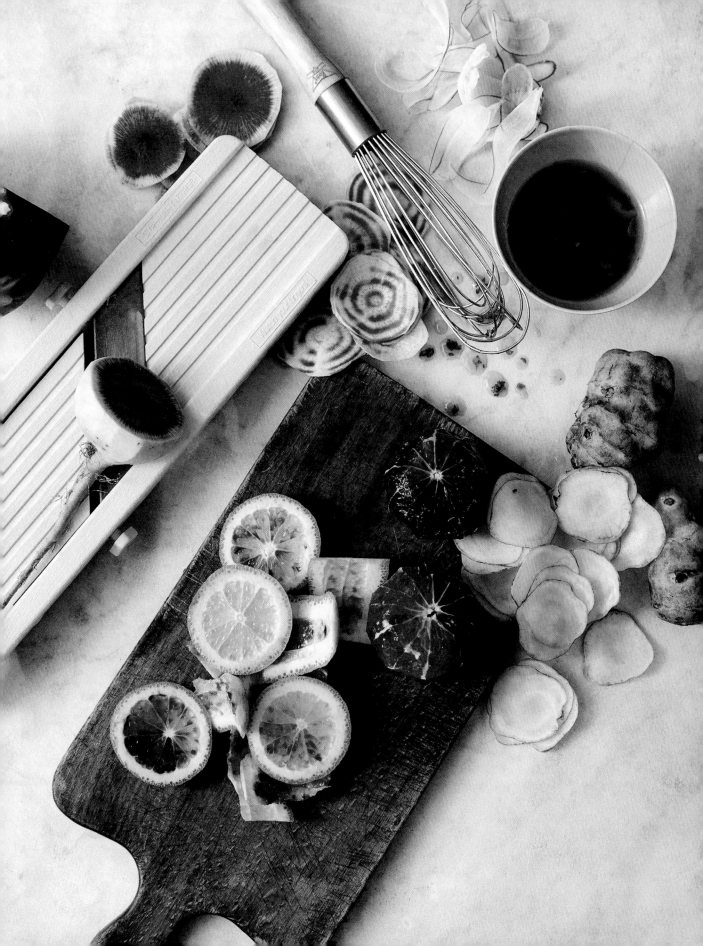

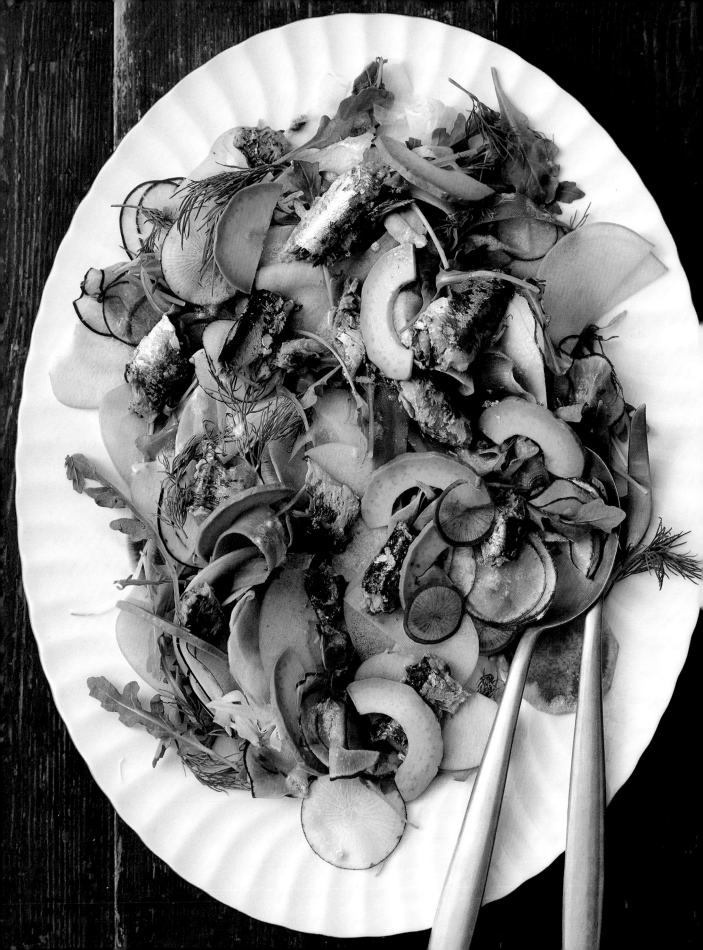

This salad is a probiotic powerhouse. A ton of fibrous vegetables get slicked with a good bacteria–rich kefir dressing. You can skip the sardines to make this a side salad, but keep them for a super-satisfying meal.

SERVES
4 TO 6

SHAVED VEGETABLE AND ARUGULA SALAD WITH KEFIR-CHIA VINAIGRETTE AND SARDINES

2 bunches medium radishes, preferably one red and one Easter Egg

3 large radishes, preferably a mix of black and watermelon

I fennel bulb

I carrot

I small rutabaga, peeled

I shallot

I tart apple, cored

I cup baby arugula

I avocado, pitted, peeled, and thinly sliced

Fresh basil, mint, and dill leaves, torn

Jacobsen flake finishing sea salt and freshly ground black pepper

Kefir-Chia Vinaigrette (recipe follows)

I (4-ounce) tin wild-caught sardines packed in olive oil, fillets cut into I-inch pieces

I lemon

Cut all the radishes, the fennel, carrot, rutabaga, shallot, and apple into paper-thin slices with a mandoline. Transfer to a large bowl and add the arugula, avocado, and herbs. Season with salt and pepper and drizzle with the vinaigrette. Toss until everything is evenly coated.

Divide among serving plates and top evenly with the sardines. Zest the lemon directly on top and serve immediately.

RECIPE CONTINUES ▶

KEFIR-CHIA VINAIGRETTE MAKES ABOUT ¾ CUP

Chia seeds soften in a tangy kefir mix, giving this dressing creaminess and lots of beneficial omega-3 fatty acids. It's especially good with crunchy shaved vegetables.

¼ cup extra-virgin olive oil

Juice of 1 lemon

½ garlic clove, grated on a Microplane

2 tablespoons white wine vinegar

¼ cup plain full-fat kefir

½ teaspoon Dijon mustard

1 teaspoon chia seeds

Coarse sea salt and freshly ground black pepper

Combine the olive oil, lemon juice, garlic, vinegar, kefir, mustard, chia, and a pinch each of salt and pepper in a jar. Seal and shake until very well combined. Season with salt and pepper.

KEFIR

Kefir is a fermented milk drink not unlike yogurt. It's made by combining milk from cows, goats, sheep, or even coconuts with kefir "grains," or bacterial cultures. Much like traditional yogurt, kefir is a living food with active live cultures, making it a terrific probiotic ingredient. I use it a lot both on its own and as an ingredient in dressings, soups, sauces, and smoothies. My favorite kefir is made by Lifeway, a family-owned company run by my friend Julie Smolyansky. I always opt for plain full-fat kefir.

This is some no-joke brain and body food! You've got tons of healthy fats from avocado and egg, anchovies for brain function, fibrous kohlrabi for gut health, and ginger and garlic for immune function and to cool inflammation. This is also seriously delicious and filling enough to be a meal on its own.

SERVES
2 TO 4

SHAVED KOHLRABI WITH SMASHED AVOCADO, ANCHOVIES, AND BOILED EGGS

I soft avocado, pitted and peeled

I tablespoon thinly sliced serrano chiles

I tablespoon grated peeled fresh ginger

¼ garlic clove, grated on a Microplane

2 cilantro sprigs, coarsely chopped

2 anchovy fillets

4 tablespoons avocado oil, plus more for drizzling

2 limes

2 kohlrabi, cut into paper-thin slices on a mandoline

Jacobsen flake finishing sea salt

2 Just-Right Boiled Eggs (page 306), peeled and halved

In a large bowl, combine the avocado, chiles, ginger, garlic, cilantro, anchovies, 2 tablespoons of the avocado oil, and the juice of 1 lime and mash together with a potato masher.

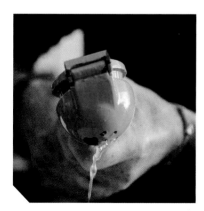
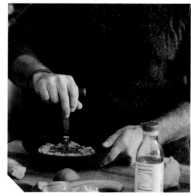
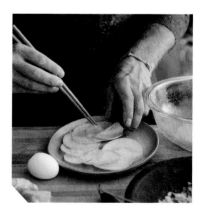

RECIPE CONTINUES ▶

2   In another large bowl, toss the kohlrabi, the juice of ½ lime, the remaining 2 tablespoons avocado oil, and a pinch of salt. Arrange on a serving plate and top with the avocado mixture and the halved eggs.

3   Zest the remaining lime half on top, sprinkle with salt, and drizzle with oil.

KOHLRABI

I like kohlrabi a lot. It has a cool apple-y flavor and it's not gassy like a turnip. You can shave it to eat raw or to pickle or cut it into chunks and roast it. Be sure to buy kohlrabi that feels firm. Soft ones won't be as fresh and crisp.

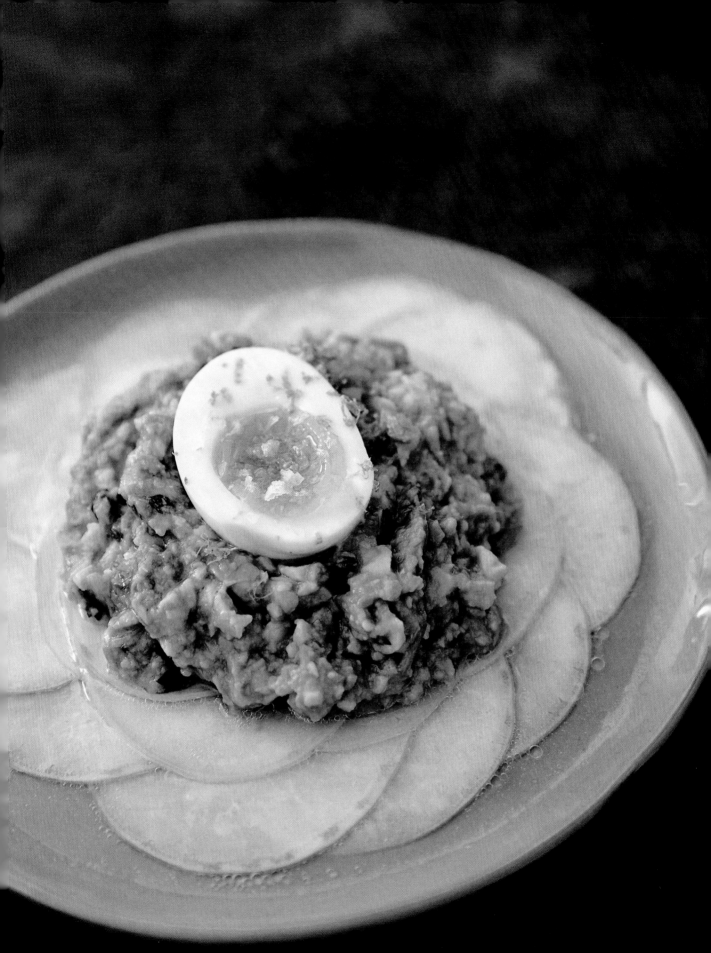

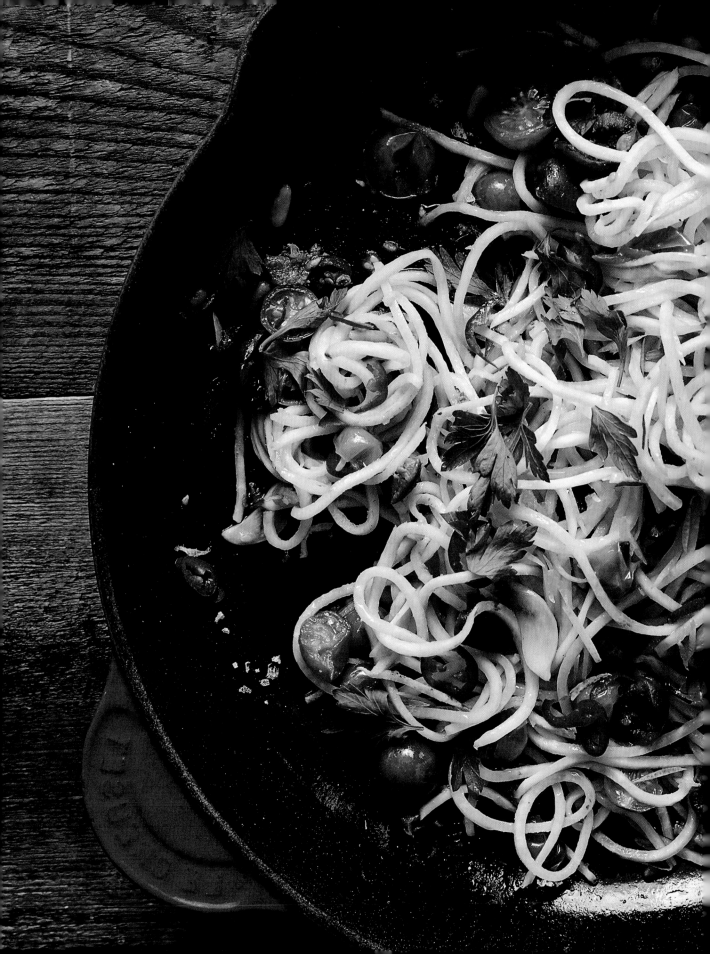

VEGETABLES

To make your body the best it can be, you need to take in tons of vegetables. The easiest way to do that is to make them so delicious, you can't stop eating them. I love cooked vegetables as much as salads, and I don't relegate them to side dish status. Instead of treating them as something to accompany meat, I make them the center of the meal. Sometimes, I'll cook and serve a bunch of small vegetable dishes and be totally satisfied. Maybe that comes from having run restaurants that serve small-plate Spanish tapas, but I promise you, it's an awesome way to eat. And it doesn't take longer than pulling together a traditional three-course meal. By shaking up the conventions of how we eat, we can achieve our goals of better health.

My tips for preparing vegetables are scattered throughout this chapter where they apply. My general guidelines are pretty straightforward and easy to follow:

- Buy the best—ideally, organic from your garden or local farmers.

- Buy a lot. Vegetables don't keep forever, so keeping your fridge stocked with them will motivate you to cook them.

- Make a lot. Leftover vegetables make the best breakfasts and lunches.

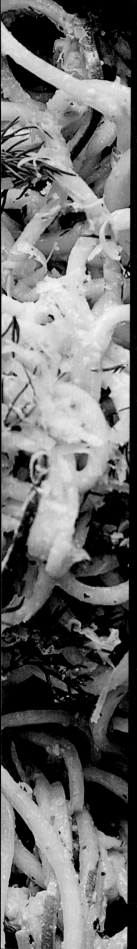

SPIRALIZE

Be wise and spiralize. My dear friends Jasmine and Melissa Hemsley of Hemsley + Hemsley are all about the spiralizer, a vegetable lathe originally from Japan that turns zucchini into pastalike strips and makes sheets out of carrots and cucumbers. It's an amazing—and amazingly easy—way to turn vegetables into unusual and interesting shapes that add whole new dimensions of texture and form to our food. It may be all the rage now, but I first used a spiralizer in 2009 when I competed on *Iron Chef America.* Back then, I had to special order one from Japan and it cost a fortune. Now you can get one inexpensively from any cooking store or online.

The spiralizer is a great kitchen tool for creating noodlelike vegetables, so you get the satisfaction of eating pasta without consuming any grains. I'm totally opposed to substitution foods, but pasta really is comforting. The difference between wheat noodles and spiralized vegetables from a health standpoint? There's no comparison.

If you want noodles, spiralize celery root for something close to spaghetti, zucchini for linguine. I also love using the spiralizer to make ribbons of summer squash that can be blanched and shocked for a cold summer salad with crab, avocado, a little chile, and fresh herbs. Add a squeeze of juice and grating of zest from a citrus fruit, and you've got a beautiful, healthy, and delicious weekend lunch!

Eating this dish reminds me of being in Sicily. The umami of anchovies with buttery pine nuts and olive oil makes the tomato blend taste like it contains cheese even though it doesn't. Celery root looks like traditional pasta (see photo on page 96) and is surprising and unexpected in a good way. Its light anise scent carries the savory topping well.

SERVES
2 TO 4

CELERY ROOT NOODLES WITH SUN GOLD TOMATOES, ANCHOVIES, AND BASIL

¼ cup extra-virgin olive oil, plus more if needed

2 tablespoons pine nuts

I small celery root, peeled and spiralized

3 anchovies in olive oil, cut into ½-inch pieces

I garlic clove, very thinly sliced

8 Castelvetrano olives, crushed, pitted, and torn

¾ cup grape or cherry tomatoes, preferably Sun Golds, halved

¼ Fresno chile, seeded, if desired, and thinly sliced

Jacobsen flake finishing sea salt

I lemon

Fresh flat-leaf parsley and basil, chopped

1 In a large cast-iron skillet, combine the olive oil and pine nuts. Cook over high heat, stirring once, until the nuts are golden, about 3 minutes. Add the celery root and anchovies and cook, stirring, for 15 seconds. Add the garlic and cook, stirring, for 1 minute.

2 Add the olives, tomatoes, and chile and stir well. Season with salt. Remove from the heat and divide among serving plates.

3 Zest the lemon directly on top and garnish with parsley and basil.

Barely cooked zucchini noodles taste almost like al dente pasta. Their subtlety benefits from a punchy pesto, salty cheese, and aromatic dill.

ZUCCHINI NOODLES WITH GARLIC SCAPE AND PISTACHIO PESTO

Kosher salt

2 medium zucchini, spiralized into spaghetti-like noodles or julienned lengthwise

¼ cup Garlic Scape and Pistachio Pesto (page 293)

Parmesan cheese

Dill leaves

Jacobsen flake finishing sea salt

Extra-virgin olive oil

1　Bring a large saucepan of generously salted water to a boil. Fill a large bowl with generously salted water and ice. Drop the zucchini into the boiling water, let it sit for 5 seconds, and transfer to the ice water. When cold, lift it into a salad spinner. Spin dry.

2　Put the noodles in a large bowl and drizzle the pesto on top. Gently toss with chopsticks until the noodles are evenly coated.

3　Divide between serving plates. Grate Parmesan on top, then scatter with dill and finishing sea salt. Drizzle with olive oil and serve immediately.

TECHNIQUE TIP: I love cooking vegetables over gentle heat in the summer. I'll throw a dried chile, thyme, and lemon peel into olive oil in a skillet and heat it over medium-low before adding some cherry tomatoes, summer squash, and snap peas. Gently sweating the vegetables without letting them brown keeps the colors bright and the flavor and texture super light and delicate. Crack a few fresh eggs into the pan and delicately scramble, and you've got a perfect lunch or breakfast. Keep the heat low and the cooking slow!

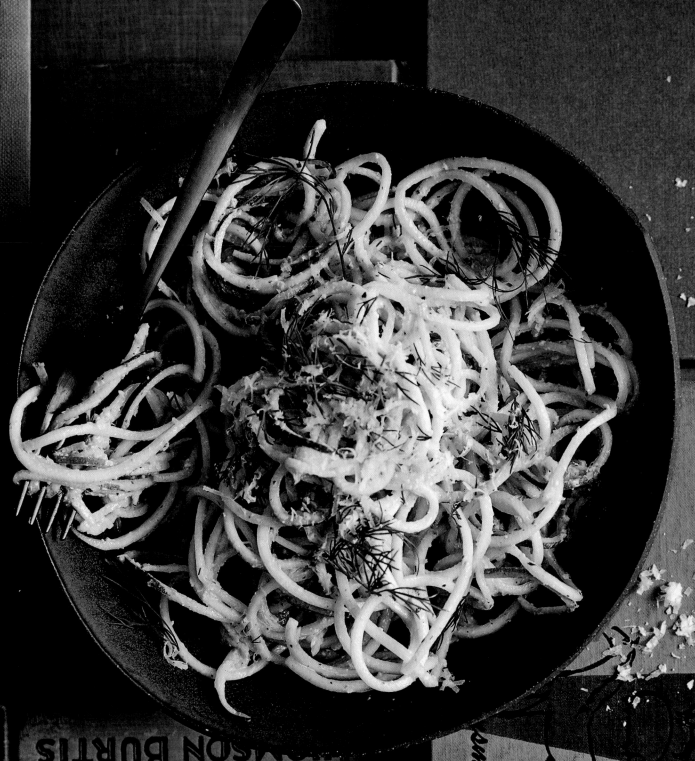

To make sure all the vegetables end up perfectly crisp-tender, I keep them the same size. But I do like to cut them into different shapes. That makes the dish more attractive and, I think, tastier. I serve this spring sauté with Perfectly Pan-Roasted Salmon (page 182).

SERVES 4

SAUTÉED ASPARAGUS, SPRING ONIONS, ARTICHOKES, AND GREENS

2 artichoke hearts, prepped (see page 38) and cut into ½-inch wedges

Extra-virgin olive oil

4 spring onions, whites halved, greens and pale green parts very thinly sliced

1 king oyster mushroom, halved lengthwise and cut into ½-inch slices crosswise

6 asparagus spears, tips kept whole, stalks cut into 2-inch lengths

1 small shallot, very thinly sliced

1 cup dandelion or other bitter tender greens, torn

2 tablespoons grass-fed unsalted butter

Coarse sea salt and freshly ground black pepper

1 teaspoon champagne vinegar

Fresh dill leaves, torn

1   Heat a large cast-iron skillet over medium-high heat. Drain the artichokes and press dry with paper towels. Coat the hot pan with a thin layer of olive oil and add the artichokes. Cook, stirring occasionally, until lightly browned, about 2 minutes.

2   Add the spring onion whites and cook, stirring often, for 2 minutes. Add the mushroom and cook, stirring, for 1 minute. Add the asparagus and cook, stirring, until bright green and crisp-tender, about 3 minutes.

3   Add the shallot, sliced spring onion greens, dandelion greens, and the butter. Season everything with salt and pepper, then cook, stirring and shaking the skillet, for 1 minute. Add the vinegar and cook, stirring, for 1 minute. Remove from the heat and top with dill. Serve immediately.

I'm not too precious about vegetables. I don't want to be fancy and bright and vibrant for the sake of being fancy and bright and vibrant. I do it for the taste. Here mustard greens are simply sautéed with only a few ingredients: garlic, anchovies, chile, and lemon. Talk about nutrient density! The dish ends up being so delicious and so nourishing.

SAUTÉED MUSTARD GREENS WITH ANCHOVIES

I bunch mustard greens, stems and leaves separated	½ garlic clove, sliced paper-thin	Pinch of Calabrian chile or red pepper flakes
Extra-virgin olive oil	Jacobsen flake finishing sea salt	Juice of ¼ lemon
	6 anchovies, cut into ½-inch pieces	

Cut the mustard green stems into ½-inch slices crosswise and cut the leaves into 3-inch slices.

Heat a large, deep skillet over medium-high heat. Coat the bottom of the skillet with olive oil. Add the mustard green stems and cook, stirring, for 1 minute. Add the mustard green leaves and stir until wilted, about 1 minute.

Add the garlic and cook, stirring occasionally, until the greens exude their water, about 3 minutes. Season with salt. Add the anchovies and chile and stir well for 2 minutes. It's okay if the anchovies break up.

Add the lemon juice and cook, stirring, for 1 minute. Remove from the heat and serve immediately.

A splash of vinegar brings out the earthiness of mushrooms and the sweetness of the greens. The combination is fantastic with Perfectly Grilled Lamb Loin Chops (page 229). Nestle the meat right into the vegetables so they soak up all the fatty juices.

SERVES
2 TO 4

SAUTÉED MAITAKE MUSHROOMS AND MUSTARD GREENS

2 tablespoons extra-virgin olive oil

4 ounces maitake mushrooms, cut into ½-inch pieces

I shallot, thinly sliced

5 garlic cloves, thinly sliced

I bunch mustard greens, ribs and stems removed, leaves torn into pieces

I tablespoon white balsamic vinegar

Jacobsen flake finishing sea salt and freshly ground black pepper

1 In a large skillet, heat the olive oil over medium-high heat. Add the mushrooms and cook, stirring occasionally, until well browned, about 4 minutes. Transfer to a plate.

2 Reduce the heat to medium and add the shallot and garlic to the skillet. Cook, stirring occasionally, until the shallot is softened and starting to brown, about 2 minutes.

3 Add the greens and season with salt and pepper. Cook, stirring occasionally, until wilted and bright green, about 2 minutes. Return the mushrooms to the skillet and toss to combine. Stir in the vinegar. Season with salt and pepper and serve immediately.

Tart dried fruit brings an acidic punch to the happy marriage of shiitakes and bok choy. Serve this with Perfect Pan-Roasted Chicken Breast (page 205) for a simple weeknight meal.

STIR-FRIED BOK CHOY AND SHIITAKES

2 tablespoons extra-virgin olive oil

10 shiitake mushrooms, stemmed, caps cut into ¼-inch slices

2 large bok choy, green kept whole, stems thinly sliced

I shallot, very thinly sliced

Jacobsen flake finishing sea salt and freshly ground black pepper

¼ cup dried golden berries or tart cherries

I teaspoon white balsamic vinegar

Heat a large skillet over medium-high heat. Add the olive oil and swirl to coat the bottom of the pan, then add the mushrooms and bok choy stems. Cook, stirring, until lightly browned and just tender, about 2 minutes.

Reduce the heat to medium and add the shallot. Cook, stirring, until just tender, about 2 minutes. Season the vegetables with salt and pepper and cook, stirring, for 2 minutes more. Add the golden berries and cook, stirring, for 3 minutes. Tear in the bok choy greens and fold in gently. Cook, stirring, just until the greens wilt, about 1 minute. Stir in the vinegar and remove from the heat. Season with salt and serve immediately.

DRIED GOLDEN BERRIES

Golden berries, also known as cape gooseberries, come from South America. When dried, they're more tart than sweet and as chewy as dried sour cherries (which make a good substitute if you can't find golden berries). In addition to having antioxidants, they also have anti-inflammatory properties.

Imagine the best sushi rice you've ever tasted, amped up with shallot, coconut, and greens. I infuse the chewy grains with tangy dressing and rich coconut oil and coconut flakes. You can top this with grilled steak for a big meal or quadruple the vegetables to make it a light lunch.

MAKES
ABOUT
2 CUPS

BABY BOK CHOY WITH COCONUT FORBIDDEN BLACK RICE

½ cup black rice

1 tablespoon jarred yuzu or fresh lime juice

5 tablespoons coconut oil

2 teaspoons minced shallot

2 teaspoons rice vinegar

2 teaspoons dried unsweetened coconut flakes

Coarse sea salt and freshly ground black pepper

4 baby bok choy, steamed and halved

Fresh cilantro

1 Cook the rice according to the package directions. In a small bowl, whisk the yuzu juice with 1 tablespoon of the coconut oil. Set aside.

2 In a large saucepan, heat 2 tablespoons of the oil over medium heat. Add the shallot and cook, stirring, until translucent. Add the vinegar and cook, stirring, until it evaporates and glazes the shallot. Add the rice and the remaining 2 tablespoons oil and fold until well mixed. Fold in the coconut flakes, then season with salt and pepper. Transfer to serving bowls, top with the bok choy and cilantro, and drizzle with the yuzu mixture. Serve immediately.

HEALTH TIP: I feel we don't really need to have grains in our lives from an evolutionary standpoint. That said, there's something very comforting about rice. I don't make it a regular part of my diet, but I also don't think there's anything wrong with consuming it periodically. I actually eat more white rice than brown rice because it has less sugar and it tends to be easier to digest. But the rice I really like is black rice, for its chewy texture, nutrients, and fiber.

Use whichever squash look best at the market—pattypan and whatnot. Any variety will taste great with the trio of aromatics: sweet leeks, peppery scapes, and sharp garlic. I Microplane the garlic so tiny bits cling to the vegetables, adding a pronounced but not overpowering fragrance. The resulting dish ends up tasting very Asian, almost like tom yum soup. It's especially good with fish, such as Perfectly Pan-Roasted Salmon (page 182) or Perfectly Grilled Halibut (page 188).

SERVES 2 TO 4

WILTED SUMMER SQUASH WITH GARLIC SCAPES, LEEKS, AND HERBS

Extra-virgin olive oil

2 small summer squash, such as zucchini and pattypan, cut into ¾-inch chunks

2 small leeks, white and pale green parts only, very thinly sliced

2 tablespoons grass-fed unsalted butter

Coarse sea salt

2 small garlic cloves, grated on a Microplane

I small serrano chile, very thinly sliced and seeded if desired

4 teaspoons very thinly sliced garlic scapes or scallions

I lemon

¼ cup fresh cilantro

Heat a large deep skillet over medium heat. Coat the bottom of the skillet with olive oil. When it shimmers, add the squash in a single layer. Cook, stirring, for just a suggestion of color and not more than that, about 1 minute.

Add the leeks and butter and season with salt. Cook, stirring, for 1 minute. Add the garlic and cook, stirring, for 2 minutes. Add the chile and garlic scapes and stir well. Zest the lemon directly on top, then halve the lemon and squeeze in the juice from one half. Remove from the heat and add the cilantro.

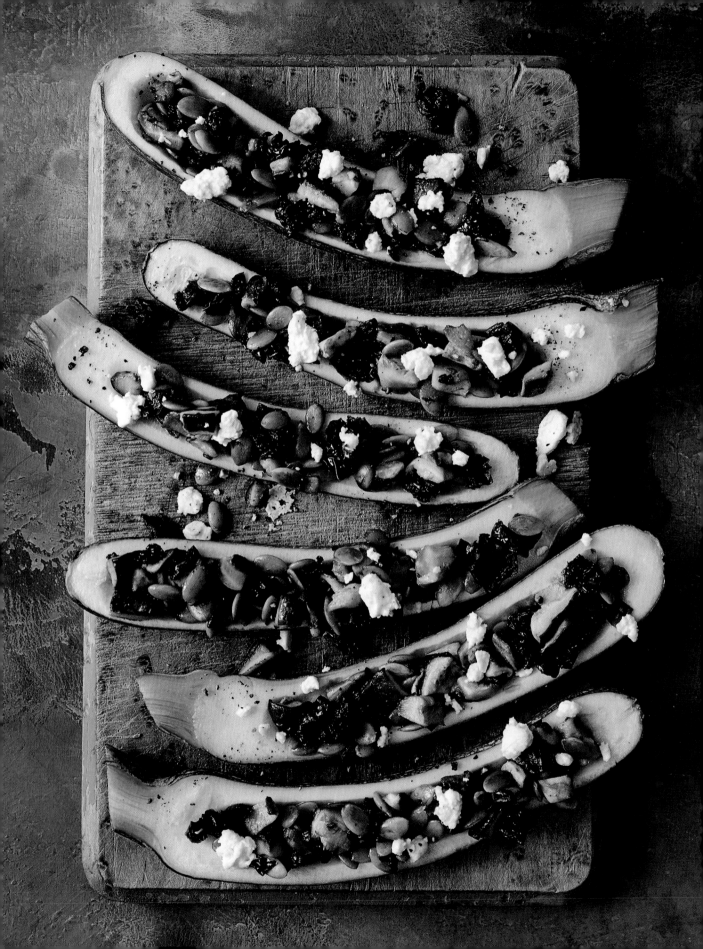

I could lie to you and tell you this is a Mexican dish. Maybe you'd even believe it. But the truth is that it's Mexican only in my mind's eye (or, more accurately, mouth). It's what I imagine food to taste like—what I want it to taste like—in Mexico. Garlicky tomatoes and mushrooms with the heat of chiles and the freshness of limes and cilantro get the toasty crunch of pepitas. Baked in summer squash boats, the mix becomes an elegant vegetarian main dish.

SERVES
2 TO 4

SUMMER SQUASH STUFFED WITH MUSHROOMS, PEPITAS, AND GOAT CHEESE

2 long slender summer squash, such as zucchini or yellow squash

Jacobsen flake finishing sea salt

Extra-virgin olive oil

2 limes

12 fresh shiitake mushrooms, stemmed, caps cut into 1/4-inch slices

5 sun-dried tomatoes, very thinly sliced

1 garlic clove, cut into thin slivers

3 tablespoons pepitas (hulled pumpkin seeds)

1/2 red finger chile, seeded, if desired, very thinly sliced

1/2 cup fresh cilantro, chopped

2 ounces goat cheese

1 Preheat the oven to 400°F.

2 Cut the squash in half lengthwise. Use a spoon to scoop out the seeds and create boats with 1/3 inch of flesh all around the edges. Set the squash on a rimmed baking sheet, cut-sides up. Sprinkle salt all over the squash, then drizzle with olive oil. Zest the limes on top.

3 Roast the squash for 10 minutes.

RECIPE CONTINUES ▶

4   Meanwhile, heat a large skillet over medium-high heat. Lightly coat the bottom of the pan with olive oil. Add the mushrooms, stir well, then add the sun-dried tomatoes. Cook, stirring, for 30 seconds, then add the garlic. Add more oil if the pan looks dry; the mushrooms have a tendency to soak up the oil. Cook, stirring, for 1 minute.

5   Add the pepitas and cook, stirring, for 1 minute, then add the chile and a big pinch of salt. Stir well, then remove from the heat. Squeeze in the juice of 1 lime and stir well, then stir in the cilantro.

6   Divide the mixture among the roasted squash cavities. Return to the oven and roast just to heat through and meld the flavors a bit, 2 to 4 minutes. You want the squash to still have a little crunch.

7   Crumble the goat cheese on top and serve immediately.

GRILLED ZUCCHINI PLANKS WITH PESTO

All summer long, I get on my deck and grill zucchini over a super-hot fire. The heat gives it a nice char while keeping the center crisp and juicy. Simply cut zucchini into 1/2-inch-thick planks, generously season with salt and pepper, coat with olive oil, and grill, turning occasionally, until grill marks appear and the zucchini is just tender. As soon as the zucchini comes off the grill, slather it with Garlic Scape and Pistachio Pesto (page 293). You can finish it off with shaved Parmesan, a drizzle of olive oil, Jacobsen flake finishing sea salt, and torn herbs.

When spaghetti squash is cooked, its flesh can be forked into capellini-like strands. The vegetable is subtle—bordering on bland—so I load it with hard-hitting seasonings while it's still hot and ready to soak up spice, sweetness, and tang. This makes a great side dish on its own or can be used as the base for Spaghetti Squash Stuffed with Ginger-Garlic Beef (page 250).

SERVES 4 TO 8

HARISSA ROASTED SPAGHETTI SQUASH

I spaghetti squash, halved lengthwise and seeded Jacobsen flake finishing sea salt	Extra-virgin olive oil 2 tablespoons harissa, plus more to taste	2 tablespoons raw honey 2 tablespoons white balsamic vinegar

1 Preheat the oven to 400°F.

2 Put the squash cut-sides up on a rimmed baking sheet. Generously season with salt and drizzle with olive oil. Divide the harissa between the squash halves and rub all over to evenly coat. Drizzle the honey all over the squash.

3 Roast until very tender, about 50 minutes.

4 Let the squash cool a bit, then run a fork all over the cut sides to lift out and separate the spaghetti-like strands of the flesh. If you need to hold the squash in place, do so with tongs or hold on to them with a kitchen towel. Transfer the flesh to a large bowl.

5 Aggressively season the squash with salt and drizzle with olive oil. Toss with the fork and drizzle with the vinegar. Add more harissa if you'd like and toss again. Serve hot.

Briny caper berries add a salty-sour punch to my take on caponata. It's good enough to eat by the spoonful, but I also like to nestle Pan-Seared Mackerel (page 191) in the hot mix during the last minute or so of cooking for a one-pan dinner.

FRESH AND DRIED TOMATO CAPONATA

1 medium Japanese eggplant, cut into 1-inch chunks

Kosher salt

¼ cup extra-virgin olive oil, plus more for serving

1 red bell pepper, thinly sliced

2 shallots, thinly sliced

3 sun-dried tomatoes, thinly sliced

1 cup grape or cherry tomatoes

2 garlic cloves, thinly sliced

1 red finger chile, seeded, if desired, and thinly sliced

4 caper berries, stemmed and thinly sliced

2 tablespoons pine nuts

2 tablespoons golden raisins

3 anchovy fillets, chopped (optional)

2 tablespoons white balsamic vinegar

2 tablespoons fresh basil, torn

2 tablespoons fresh tarragon, torn

1 tablespoon very thinly sliced fresh sage leaves

1 lemon

1 Sprinkle the eggplant generously with the salt and let sit for 10 minutes to get rid of any bitterness. Rinse well, then pat dry with paper towels.

2 Heat a large skillet over medium-high heat. Add the olive oil and swirl to coat the bottom of the skillet. When the oil is hot but not smoking, add the eggplant, pepper, shallots, sun-dried tomatoes, and fresh tomatoes. Generously season with salt and cook, stirring often, until the vegetables are just tender, about 5 minutes. Reduce the heat if the vegetables are browning too much before softening.

3 Add the garlic and chile and reduce the heat to low if you haven't already. Cook, stirring often, until the vegetables are very soft, about 15 minutes.

Add the caper berries, pine nuts, raisins, and anchovies (if using). Stir well, then add the vinegar. Cook, stirring and crushing the tomatoes occasionally, until the whole mixture cooks down, about 8 minutes.

Remove from the heat and stir in the basil, tarragon, and sage. You want the herbs to melt into it. Season with salt. When ready to serve, transfer to a serving plate and zest the lemon directly on top, then drizzle with oil.

SUN-DRIED TOMATOES

They were trendy in the nineties, but faded from use over the years. I actually forgot about them until I used them again while in Italy. I like the intensity of the dry-packed (not in oil) kind. They hydrate as they cook, but retain a concentrated tartness and chew.

Using a whole broccoli head, crown to stem, gives you even more fiber and nutrients, plus a duo of crunch and tenderness. Since the stems can be bland, I pickle them in the time it takes to sear the florets, and I toss the florets with the spicy vinaigrette while they're still hot. The sauce would be great on asparagus, too. If you want to turn this into a one-skillet dinner, make Seared Bone-In Smoked Pork Chops (page 257) first, then cook the broccoli in the same pan. If you do that, you don't need to salt the broccoli because the fat in the pan will be plenty salty.

SERVES
2 TO 4

BROCCOLI FLORETS WITH GOCHUJANG VINAIGRETTE AND PICKLED BROCCOLI STEMS

2 heads broccoli

½ cup plus 2 tablespoons rice vinegar

2 tablespoons gochujang

¼ cup plus 2 tablespoons coconut oil, warmed just until liquid

Jacobsen flake finishing sea salt

3 tablespoons fresh basil

3 tablespoons fresh cilantro

3 tablespoons fresh mint

Sesame seeds

1   Cut the crowns from the stems of the broccoli. Peel the stems and cut into paper-thin slices on a mandoline. Cut the crowns into small, individual florets.

2   Put the sliced stems in a bowl and pour over ½ cup of the vinegar. Let stand while preparing the florets.

3   Whisk the gochujang and remaining 2 tablespoons vinegar in a large bowl. While whisking, slowly add ¼ cup of the coconut oil in a steady stream.

4 Heat a large cast-iron skillet over high heat. Add the remaining 2 tablespoons oil and swirl to coat the bottom of the skillet. When the oil is smoking, add the broccoli florets. Cook, shaking the pan occasionally, until browned and al dente, about 5 minutes. Season with salt.

5 Add the gochujang mixture and toss well until the florets are evenly coated. Pour out the vinegar from the bowl with the broccoli stems, leaving just a bit behind. Add the basil, cilantro, and mint and toss well. Scatter over the hot florets, sprinkle with sesame seeds, and serve immediately.

GOCHUJANG

Sweet and spicy, this Korean condiment, available at Asian markets, is made of rice or barley powder mixed with red pepper and fermented soybeans. That fermentation makes it great for gut health and gives the paste a funky richness.

Fat florets of cauliflower stay meaty when roasted. I really like this with orange or yellow cauliflower. If you happen to have pickled chiles, use them in place of the fresh chiles here.

SERVES
4 TO 6

COCONUT ROASTED CAULIFLOWER WITH CILANTRO AND LIME

I head cauliflower, leaves discarded, bottom trimmed

I tablespoon coconut oil, warmed just until liquid

Jacobsen flake finishing sea salt and freshly ground black pepper

2 tablespoons ground coriander

½ red finger chile, sliced

½ lime

Cilantro sprigs

1 Preheat the oven to 400°F.

2 Cut the cauliflower into large chunks. Put the florets in a single layer on a rimmed baking sheet.

3 Spoon the coconut oil all over the cauliflower, letting it run down the sides. Sprinkle with salt, then dust with the coriander.

4 Roast until the cauliflower is very browned on top and bottom, about 30 minutes.

5 Top with the chile and squeeze lime juice all over. Top with cilantro and season with salt and pepper. Serve hot or warm.

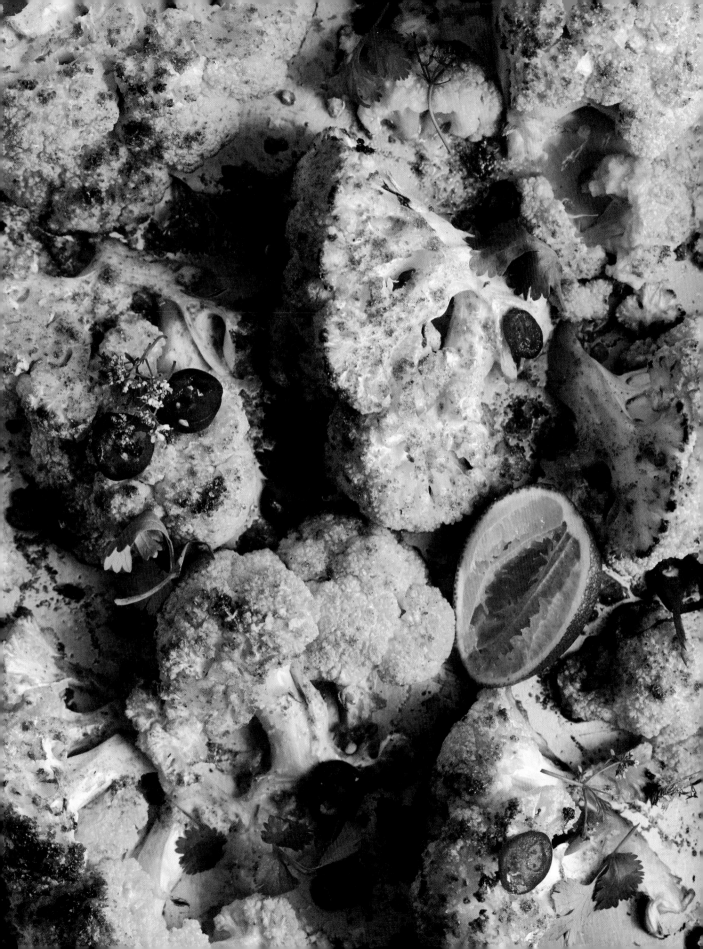

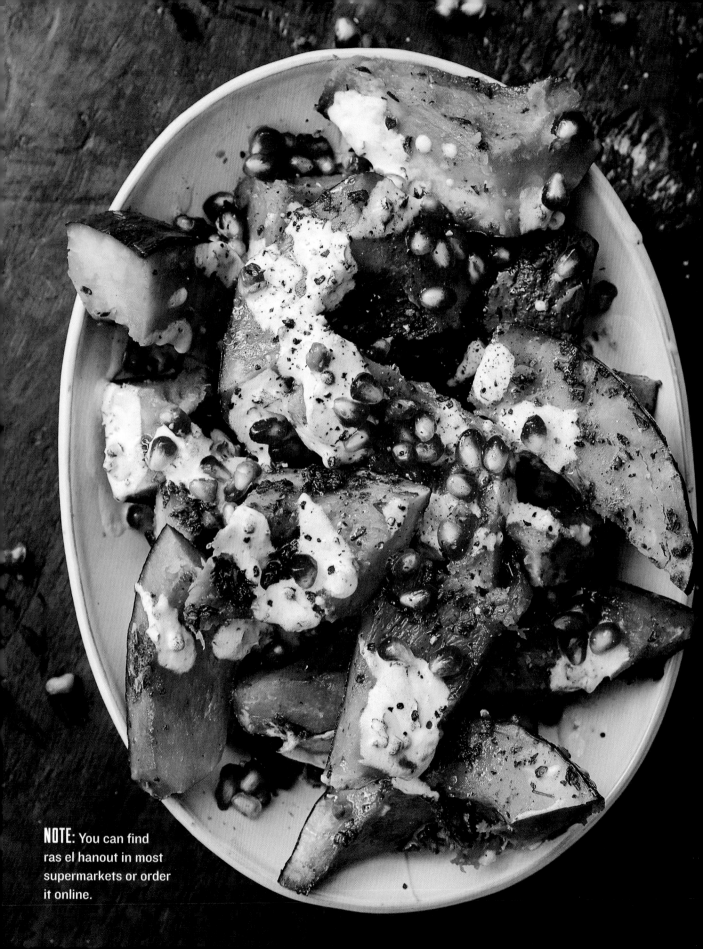

NOTE: You can find ras el hanout in most supermarkets or order it online.

A citrus-herb oil seals Moroccan ras el hanout spice to squash. *Ras el hanout* literally translates to "head of the shop," referring to how top-shelf spices are used in the mix. The warming, aromatic blend can include up to thirty spices and usually starts with at least cumin, coriander, ginger, cinnamon, nutmeg, pepper, and allspice. When the squash wedges roast, the warm seasonings soak into the flesh and create a caramelized crust.

SERVES 8

RAS EL HANOUT ROASTED KABOCHA SQUASH

I medium kabocha squash, scrubbed, halved, seeded, and cut into 8 wedges

Leaves from I small bunch sage

Leaves from I small bunch thyme

I garlic clove, grated on a Microplane

½ cup extra-virgin olive oil

Zest and juice of I orange

¼ cup pure maple syrup

I tablespoon ras el hanout spice

Jacobsen flake finishing sea salt and freshly ground black pepper

Pomegranate Yogurt Sauce (page 291)

1. Preheat the oven to 400°F.

2. In a food processor, combine the sage, thyme, garlic, oil, and orange zest and juice and process until smooth. Transfer to a bowl and whisk in the maple syrup. Arrange the squash in a single layer in a glass or ceramic baking dish. Using a pastry brush, thoroughly brush the squash with the maple-oil mixture. Sprinkle with the ras el hanout, then season with salt and pepper.

3. Cover the dish with aluminum foil and roast until the flesh and skin of the squash are tender, about 35 minutes. A paring knife should slide through easily.

4. Uncover the squash. Divide among serving dishes, top with yogurt sauce, and season with salt and pepper. Serve immediately.

There's a simplicity to this dish that's really nice. Sugary with dates caramelized in butter and salty from a final crunchy sprinkle of sea salt, gently cooked sweet potatoes become deeply comforting.

STEAMED SWEET POTATOES WITH DATE BUTTER

2 sweet potatoes, scrubbed well and cut into ½-inch-thick rounds

2 tablespoons grass-fed unsalted butter

5 Medjool dates, pitted and cut into ¼-inch dice

Jacobsen flake finishing sea salt

1 Prepare a large steamer.

2 Put the sweet potato rounds in the steamer in a single layer. Steam until tender, 12 to 15 minutes.

3 Meanwhile, combine the butter and dates in a small saucepan. Heat over medium-low heat, swirling the pan occasionally, just until the butter has melted. Remove from the heat.

4 Arrange the sweet potatoes on a serving plate in a single layer. Spoon the dates and melted butter all over, then sprinkle with salt. Serve hot or warm.

GRASS-FED BUTTER

Butter makes everything, especially vegetables, taste amazing with its creaminess. I use it moderately and I only use butter from grass-fed cows, which is now increasingly available.

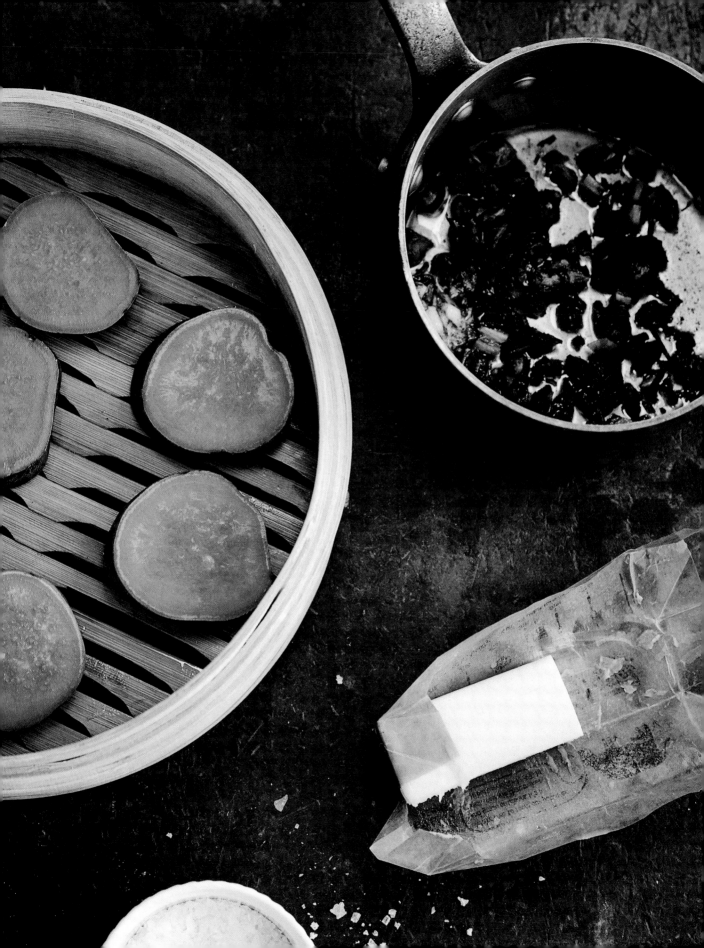

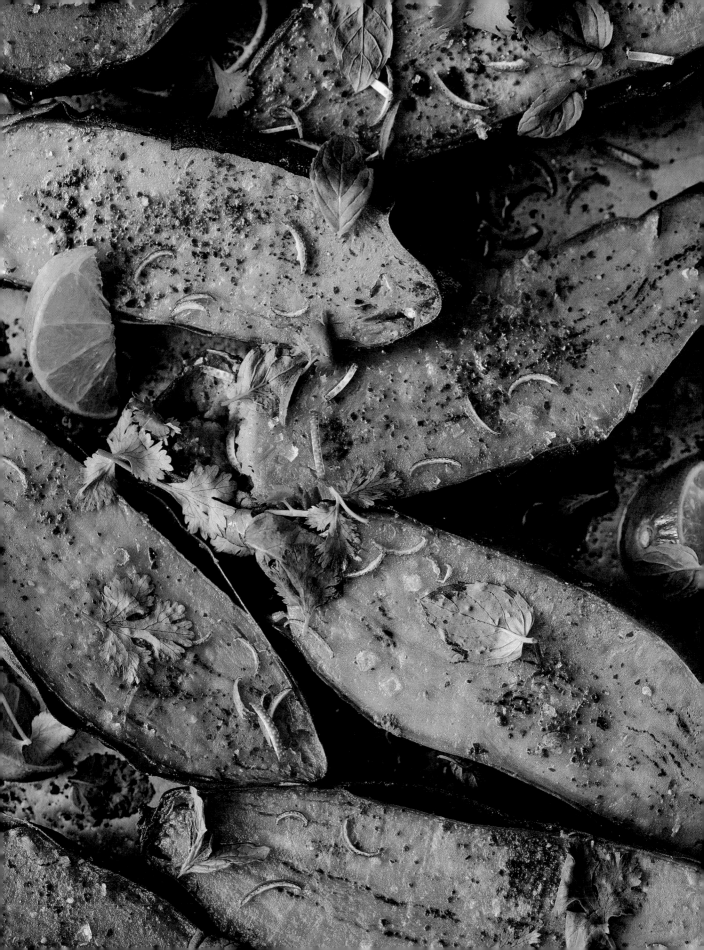

Split and slathered with coconut oil, butter, and maple syrup, sweet potatoes develop a crackly crust over their tender flesh. Salt, chile, lime, and herbs sprinkled on top catch in the crags, ensuring a hit of heat and acid in every sweet bite.

ROASTED SWEET POTATOES WITH COCONUT, MAPLE SYRUP, AND ESPELETTE PEPPER

4 medium sweet potatoes

4 tablespoons coconut oil

4 tablespoons grass-fed unsalted butter

4 teaspoons pure maple syrup

2 tablespoons Jacobsen flake finishing sea salt

2 teaspoons Espelette pepper or chile powder

Zest and juice of 1 lime

Fresh cilantro and mint leaves

1   Preheat the oven to 400°F.

2   Place the whole sweet potatoes on a roasting pan and roast until tender and cooked through, about 30 minutes. The timing will depend on their size. Remove from the oven and cut each sweet potato in half lengthwise. Return to the roasting pan, cut-sides up.

3   Change the oven setting to broil or heat the broiler. Rub the cut sides of each sweet potato half with ½ tablespoon each of the coconut oil and the butter, then drizzle with the maple syrup. Sprinkle with salt and place under the broiler. Broil until slightly browned and caramelized, 3 to 5 minutes. Finish with a sprinkle of Espelette pepper, the lime zest, lime juice, and cilantro and mint. Serve immediately.

Carrots develop big flavors when you marinate them in spices, then toss them in the same mix after a turn on the grill. The minted yogurt complements the warm seasonings and turns this into a dish worthy of being the main course.

SERVES 4

MARINATED SPICE-GRILLED CARROTS WITH MINT, YOGURT, AND PISTACHIOS

I small guindilla pepper or chile de árbol

I teaspoon coriander seeds

I teaspoon cumin seeds

I teaspoon mustard seeds

¼ teaspoon whole black peppercorns

¼ teaspoon whole cloves

½ star anise pod

2 tablespoons extra-virgin olive oil

I tablespoon sherry vinegar

I small garlic clove, finely grated

2 pounds mixed heirloom baby carrots

Jacobsen flake finishing sea salt

Mint Yogurt Sauce (page 290)

¼ cup unsalted shelled pistachios, toasted

Fresh mint leaves, torn

Aged balsamic vinegar

1   Heat a grill to medium-high.

2   In a spice grinder, combine the guindilla, coriander, cumin, mustard, peppercorns, cloves, and star anise and pulse until ground. Transfer to a large bowl and add the olive oil, sherry vinegar, and garlic. Whisk to blend. Add the carrots, season with salt, and toss until well coated. Let stand for 20 minutes. Transfer the carrots to the grill, reserving the spice oil in the bowl.

3   Grill the carrots, turning often and taking care not to burn them, until tender, 7 to 10 minutes. Return to the bowl with the spice oil. Gently toss to coat, then refrigerate until cool.

4   Place the mint yogurt in the bottom of a large bowl. Arrange the chilled carrots on top. Sprinkle with the pistachios and mint leaves and finish with a generous drizzle of the aged balsamic vinegar.

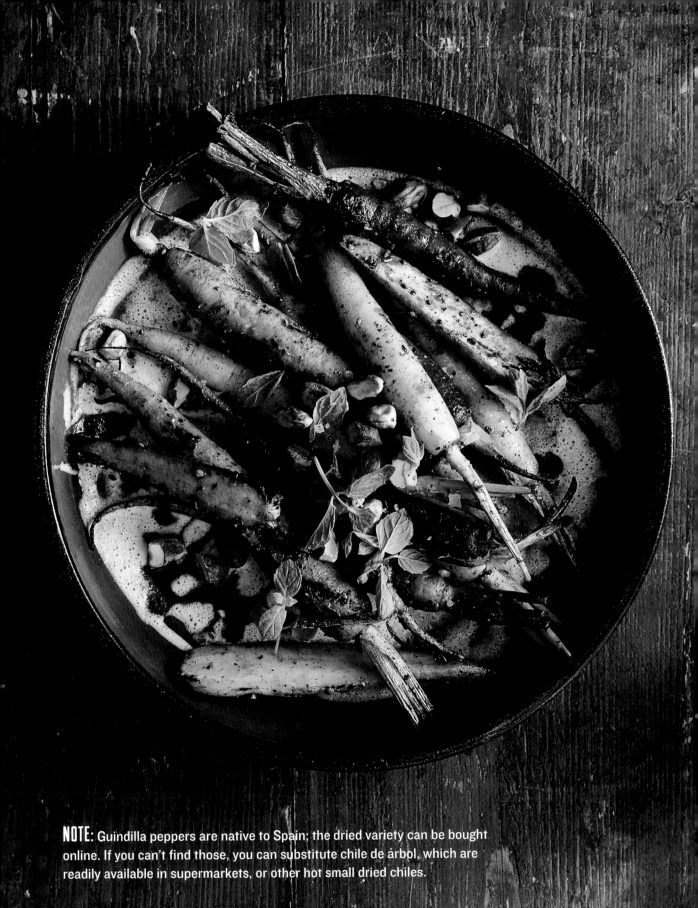

NOTE: Guindilla peppers are native to Spain; the dried variety can be bought online. If you can't find those, you can substitute chile de árbol, which are readily available in supermarkets, or other hot small dried chiles.

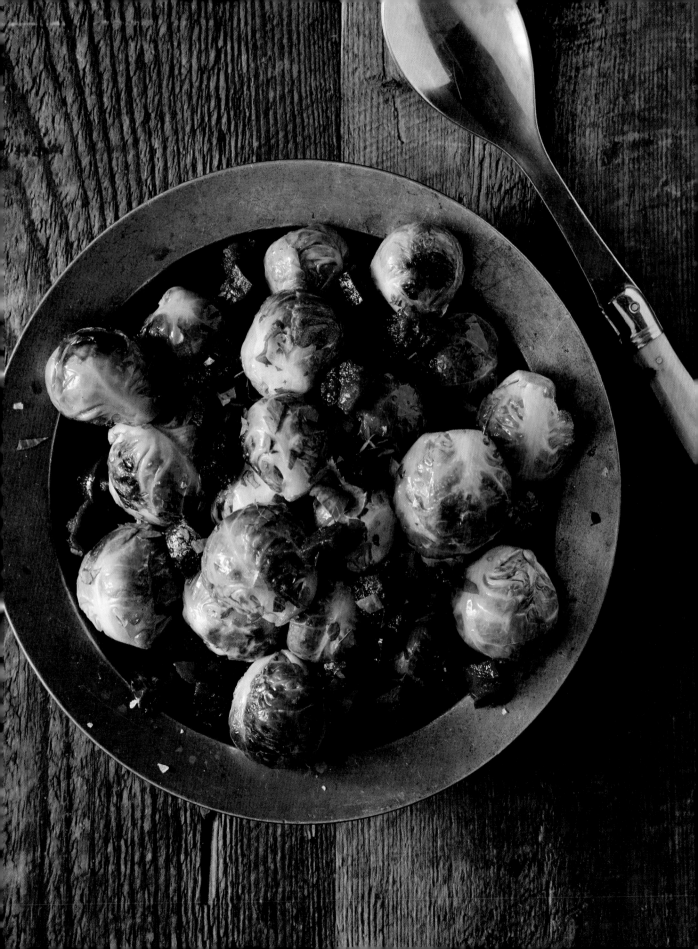

When I put roasted Brussels sprouts on my restaurant menus, the dishes fly out of the kitchen with reckless abandon. People want their sprouts! They're the meatballs of the vegetable world. Here, a little chorizo and some lemon juice go a long way to taking the boredom out of sprouts.

SERVES 4

PAN-ROASTED BRUSSELS SPROUTS

3 tablespoons extra-virgin olive oil

1 pound Brussels sprouts, preferably small

8 ounces dried chorizo, diced

1 tablespoon fresh lemon juice

1 cup Chicken Stock (page 139) or store-bought unsalted chicken broth

Jacobsen flake finishing sea salt and freshly ground black pepper

2 tablespoons chopped fresh flat-leaf parsley

1. Heat a large cast-iron pan over medium-high heat. Add the olive oil and swirl to coat the bottom of the pan. Add the Brussels sprouts and cook, shaking the pan occasionally to gently brown on all sides, for about 3 minutes.

2. Add the chorizo and cook, stirring often, for about 2 minutes. The sprouts will start to take on a nice rosy color from the sausage. Add the lemon juice, stock, and a pinch each of salt and pepper. Simmer until the liquid has reduced and the sprouts are tender, about 5 minutes.

3. Sprinkle with the parsley and serve immediately.

Simmering sunchokes with herbs and chile before roasting infuses them with aromatics while giving them an almost creamy tenderness. Raw sunchoke coins and toasted sunflower seeds add crunch to the roasted knobs sweetened with quince vinaigrette.

SERVES 4

ROASTED AND RAW SUNCHOKES WITH QUINCE VINAIGRETTE

I lemon, halved

2 parsley sprigs

I pound sunchokes, scrubbed

I sage sprig

I thyme sprig

I bay leaf

I dried chile

I garlic clove

Jacobsen flake finishing sea salt and freshly ground black pepper

Extra-virgin olive oil

Quince Vinaigrette (recipe follows)

I cup sunflower sprouts

2 tablespoons hulled, unsalted sunflower seeds, toasted

Fresh mint leaves, torn

1 Preheat the oven to 425°F.

2 Squeeze the lemon into a bowl of cold water and drop in the halves (this is your acidulated water). Add the parsley. Cut 2 sunchokes into paper-thin coins with a mandoline and put them in the acidulated water.

SUNCHOKES

Also known as Jerusalem artichoke, this North American root vegetable looks like ginger. Gnarly and knobby, they have paper-thin skin that can simply be scrubbed clean and ivory flesh that's crunchy when raw and creamy when cooked. It's packed with inulin, a prebiotic fiber good for boosting the immune system and keeping you full.

3 In a large saucepot, combine the sage, thyme, bay leaf, chile, garlic, 6 cups water, and ¼ cup salt. Bring to a boil, then add the remaining sunchokes. Cook until tender, about 15 minutes. A paring knife should slide through easily. Drain well and let cool slightly. Discard the aromatics.

4 When cool enough to handle, toss the blanched sunchokes with enough olive oil to coat and spread them in a single layer on a rimmed baking sheet. Roast until crisp, about 10 minutes.

5 Spread the vinaigrette on a serving platter. Top with the crisp sunchokes. Drain the raw sunchokes and scatter them on top, along with the sprouts, sunflower seeds, and mint. Serve immediately.

QUINCE VINAIGRETTE MAKES ABOUT ⅔ CUP

Membrillo, Spanish quince paste, captures the plummy essence of the fruit in a block thick enough to slice. Blended into a dressing, it becomes versatile enough to coat everything from bitter greens to root vegetables.

¼ cup quince paste

Zest and juice of 1 lemon

½ garlic clove, grated on a Microplane

¼ cup extra-virgin olive oil

1 teaspoon champagne vinegar

Jacobsen flake finishing sea salt and freshly ground black pepper

In a blender or food processor, puree the quince paste, lemon zest, lemon juice, garlic, olive oil, and vinegar until smooth. Season with salt and pepper.

The probiotics in kefir, along with the fiber of sunchokes, make this dish great for your gut. Those two ingredients work so well together here, too, with the lemony yogurt coating spice-crusted roasted sunchokes.

SERVES 4

MAPLE-ROASTED SUNCHOKES WITH KEFIR AND NIGELLA SEEDS

¼ cup pure maple syrup

¼ cup plus 2 tablespoons
   extra-virgin olive oil

I pound sunchokes, scrubbed and
   halved if large

Jacobsen flake finishing sea salt and
   freshly ground black pepper

¼ cup nigella seeds or coriander
   seeds, toasted and lightly crushed

I cup plain full-fat kefir

I garlic clove, grated on a Microplane

Zest and juice of I lemon

¼ cup fresh flat-leaf parsley,
   coarsely chopped

1 Preheat the oven to 375°F.

2 In a large bowl, whisk together the maple syrup and 2 tablespoons of the olive oil. Add the sunchokes and toss until evenly coated. Season with salt and pepper and spread in an even layer in a roasting pan. Sprinkle with the nigella seeds.

3 Roast until tender, about 30 minutes. A paring knife should slide through one easily.

4 Meanwhile, in a small bowl, whisk together the kefir, garlic, lemon zest, lemon juice, and remaining ¼ cup oil until smooth. Season with salt and pepper.

5 Transfer the kefir sauce to a bowl, top with the sunchokes, and sprinkle with the parsley. Serve immediately.

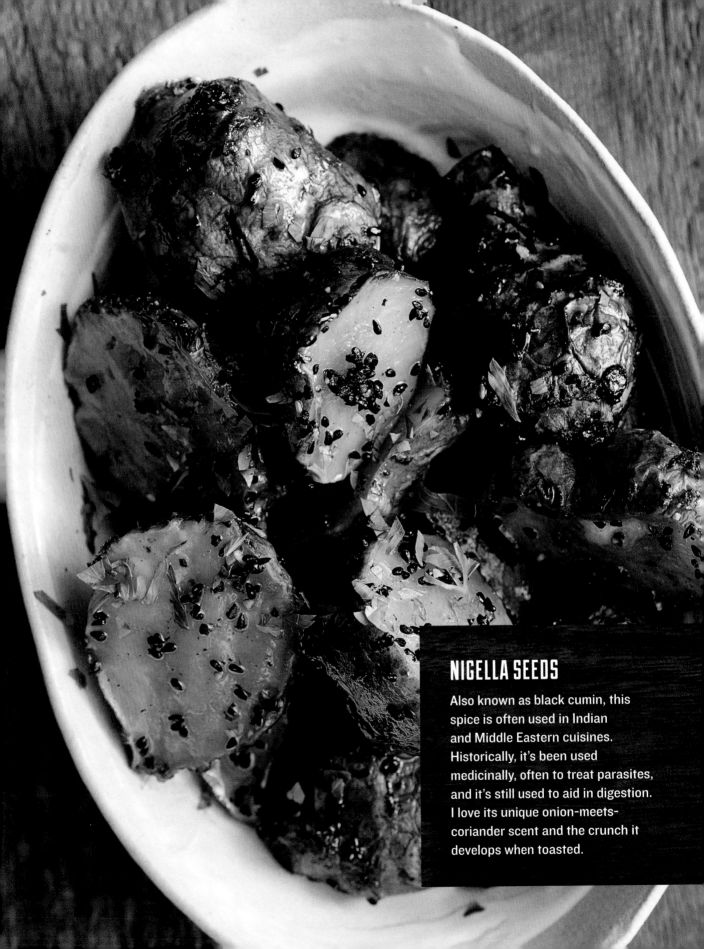

NIGELLA SEEDS

Also known as black cumin, this spice is often used in Indian and Middle Eastern cuisines. Historically, it's been used medicinally, often to treat parasites, and it's still used to aid in digestion. I love its unique onion-meets-coriander scent and the crunch it develops when toasted.

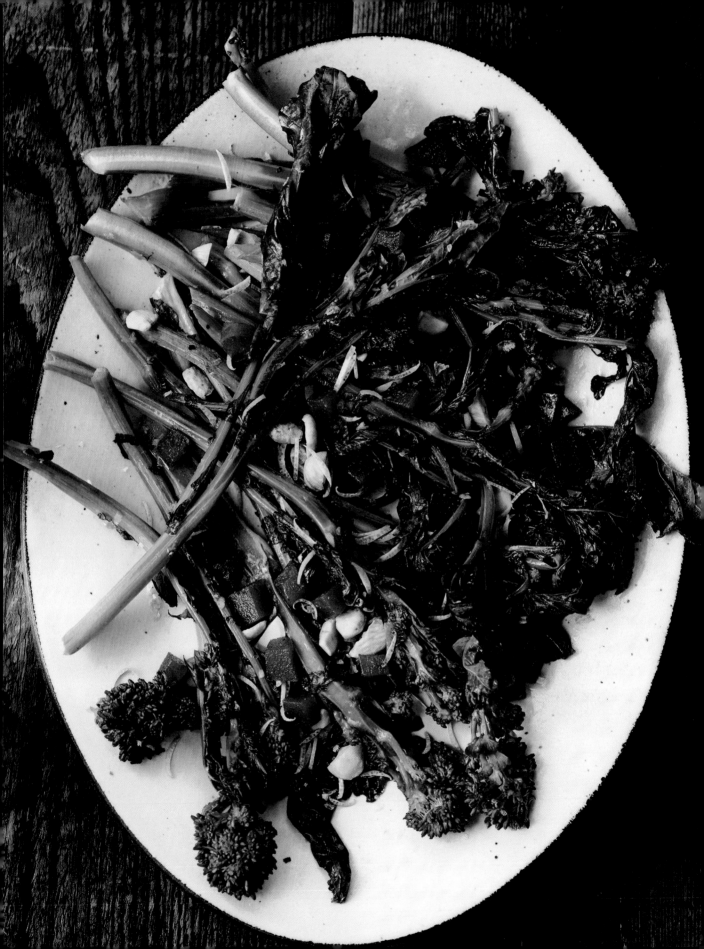

Rapini, also called broccoli rabe, is one of my all-time favorite vegetables. I'm a big fan of bitter greens and none gets me going the way rapini does. There's a natural spiciness to it, and fresh horseradish really helps bring that bite out in this dish. The sweet quince paste mellows the bitterness in a very elegant way.

SERVES 4

SPICY RAPINI WITH ALMONDS, HORSERADISH, AND QUINCE

2 tablespoons extra-virgin olive oil

2 bunches rapini, each stalk halved lengthwise

2 garlic cloves, thinly sliced

I tablespoon grated fresh horseradish

I tablespoon red pepper flakes

¼ cup Marcona almonds, coarsely chopped

Jacobsen flake finishing sea salt and freshly ground black pepper

2 tablespoons diced quince paste

Juice of I lemon

In a large skillet, heat the olive oil over medium-high heat. Add the rapini and cook, stirring, until it starts to wilt and takes on a little bit of color, about 2 minutes. Toss in the garlic, horseradish, red pepper flakes, and almonds and season with salt and pepper. Cook for 2 minutes more, then transfer to a large serving platter.

Sprinkle with the diced quince paste and lemon juice and serve immediately.

TECHNIQUE TIP: The easiest way to trim rapini stems is to cut them with kitchen shears.

Sometimes, I prefer firm, slightly underripe avocados, especially when I want to cook them. Here the grill warms avocado halves until their fat starts to melt and the fruit becomes creamy. The citrus salsa and crunchy radishes keep the dish feeling nice and light, but goat cheese crumbles on top wouldn't hurt.

SERVES 4

GRILLED AVOCADOS WITH CITRUS SALSA

2 firm avocados, halved and pitted	Jacobsen flake finishing sea salt	2 red radishes, very thinly sliced
Avocado oil	Grapefruit and Jalapeño Salsa (page 298)	

1   Heat a grill to high or heat a grill pan over high heat.

2   Trim the rounded side of each avocado half so they can sit flat without toppling.

3   Rub the cut sides of the avocados (including the trimming, if you'd like) with avocado oil to coat. Place on the grill, cut-sides down. Grill, rotating once, until cross-hatched grill marks appear and the fruit is warm all the way through, 5 to 10 minutes.

4   Place the avocados on serving plates, cut-sides up, and season with salt. Spoon the salsa on top, then scatter the radishes over all. Serve immediately.

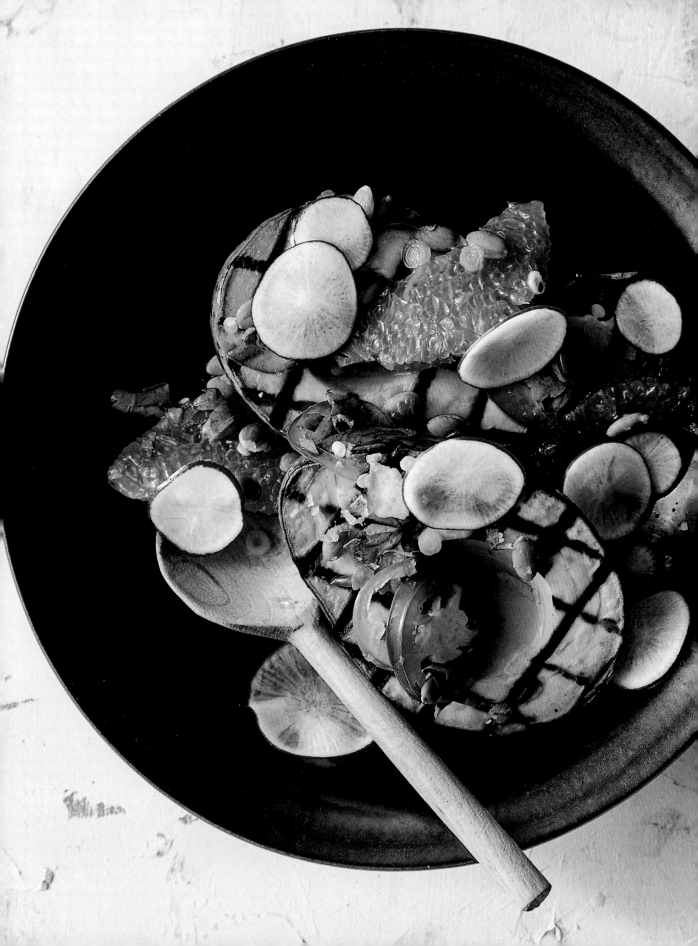

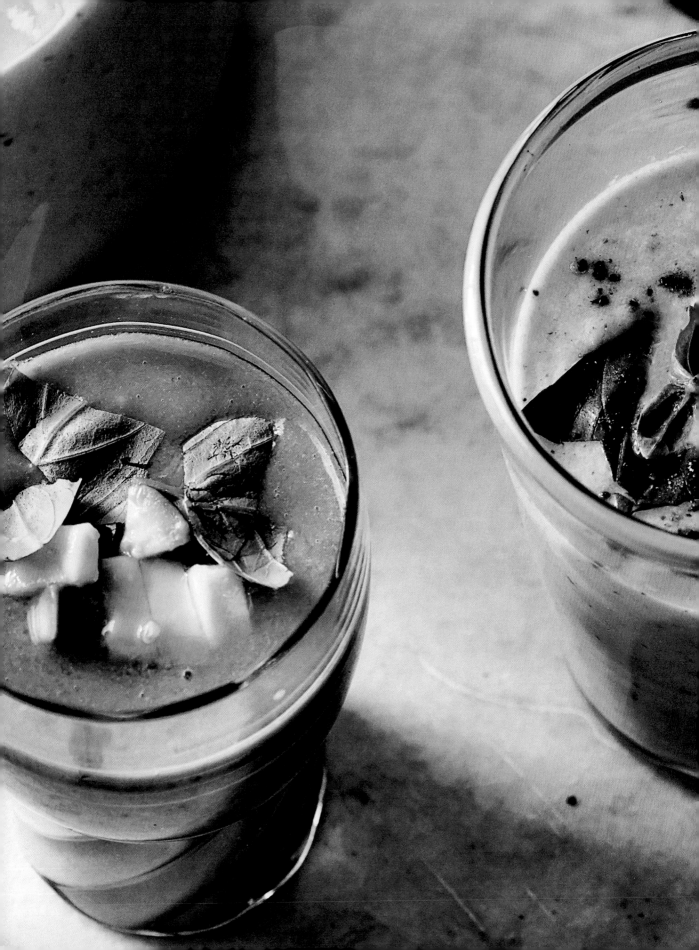

SOUPS

Soups and broths are the original medicine—and with good reason. Good bone broth and chicken stock have lots of collagen, fat, and protein, which are fundamental to a healthy gut. It's warming and easy to digest. When you add ginger, garlic, and other aromatic alliums, it becomes a kind of natural elixir that's extremely satisfying.

The bone broth craze blew up a few years ago, but all my chef friends and I have known its healing power for years. When you're feeling a little under the weather, you dip your ladle into the chicken stock simmering in every restaurant kitchen and pour yourself a nice bowl. Season it with a drop of vinegar and a pinch of salt and drink up. It's one of the heartiest and smartest things you can do to keep from getting sick.

Beyond broth, soup remains one of my favorite meals. Pureed vegetable soups have a luxurious texture, and soups chunky with produce and proteins are soothing and comforting. Soups are the secret to eating well even when you're busy. Make big batches when you're not slammed and keep them in the fridge or freezer so you can have some any time. Instead of reaching for unhealthy carb-heavy snacks when you're hungry, have a cup of soup instead. It'll fill you up and give you tons of energy.

And there are soups for every season. I grew up in Vermont, and having a hot bowl of soup was always a welcome relief from the cold after sledding. As a young adult living in southern Spain, I came to appreciate cold, refreshing *gazpacho* and *ajo blanco* during the incredibly hot summers.

In this day and age, those of us who are into food and are conscientious about the seasonality of ingredients sometimes may not realize why we gravitate toward specific dishes in different times of year. Soups are a great lens into that seasonality. Fresh produce simply tastes different whether served hot or cold. For example, a cold carrot soup may contain ginger and citrus and taste crisp and bright. A hot one with cinnamon and star anise will be warming. The effect on the palate is completely different, but the pleasure is equally great.

Stock is the secret to deep, complex flavors in soups and stews. In my vegetable version, I add butternut squash for its earthy sweetness.

VEGETABLE STOCK

2 butternut squash, peeled, seeded, and coarsely chopped

2 large carrots, cut into 2-inch pieces

2 celery stalks, cut into 2-inch pieces

I fennel bulb, cut into 2-inch pieces

6 garlic cloves

I large onion, quartered

4 thyme sprigs

Bouquet garni of whole aromatic spices, such as peppercorns, coriander, allspice, cinnamon, and clove

1   In a large stockpot, combine all the ingredients with 10 cups cold water. Bring to a boil, then reduce the heat to low and simmer, uncovered, for 1½ hours.

2   Strain through a fine-mesh sieve and discard the solids. Use immediately or transfer to airtight containers and refrigerate for up to 7 days or freeze for up to 3 months.

This is a delicious light chicken stock. For a deeper, richer flavor, try roasting the chicken carcasses in a 400°F oven until golden before simmering the stock.

MAKES
2 ½ QUARTS

CHICKEN STOCK

2 chicken carcasses

2 large carrots, cut into 2-inch pieces

2 celery stalks, cut into 2-inch pieces

I fennel bulb, cut into 2-inch pieces

6 garlic cloves

I large onion, quartered

4 thyme sprigs

Bouquet garni of whole aromatic spices, such as peppercorns, coriander, allspice, cinnamon, and clove

I cup dry white wine

2 cups dried shiitake mushrooms

1 In a large stockpot, combine all the ingredients with 10 cups cold water. Bring to a boil, then reduce the heat to low and simmer, uncovered, for 3½ to 4 hours.

2 Strain through a fine-mesh sieve and discard the solids. Use immediately or transfer to airtight containers and refrigerate for up to 7 days or freeze for up to 3 months.

I like to get a mix of shinbones and oxtails for this bone broth, but you can take whatever the butcher has. The broth will be delicious either way. I like to simmer the broth for 12 hours, which is how you end up with the 5½-quart yield. If you cook it for a shorter period of time, you'll end up with more broth. Both cooking times make big batches so I can freeze the broth in half-pint jars to reheat and sip a cup anytime. While I love to sip this broth on its own, it also makes a perfect base for soups and stews, and even for cooking flavorful quinoa or rice.

MAKES ABOUT 5½ QUARTS

ROASTED BONE BROTH WITH AROMATIC SPICES

6 pounds grass-fed beef bones

I pound carrots, cut into very large chunks

4 celery stalks, cut into very large chunks

2 onions, quartered

4 garlic cloves

I cup dried shiitake mushrooms

I (2-inch) piece fresh ginger, scrubbed and lightly crushed, plus ¼ cup grated peeled fresh ginger

¼ cup raw apple cider vinegar

I tablespoon juniper berries

I tablespoon whole black peppercorns

8 star anise pods

4 cinnamon sticks

1   Preheat the oven to 400°F. Fit a metal rack in a very large roasting pan or rimmed baking sheet.

2   Place the bones on the rack and roast, turning occasionally, until evenly golden brown, 45 minutes to 1 hour. Very carefully transfer the rack to a heatproof work surface.

3   Transfer 2 tablespoons of the rendered beef bone fat from the roasting pan to a large stockpot and set over medium-high heat. Add the carrots, celery, onions, garlic, mushrooms, and crushed ginger. Cook, stirring occasionally, until just golden, about 5 minutes.

4 Add the vinegar, roasted bones, and 14 quarts cold water. Raise the heat to high and bring to a boil. Reduce the heat to maintain a simmer and add the juniper berries, peppercorns, star anise, and cinnamon sticks.

5 For a nice, light broth, simmer for 4 to 6 hours. For a deeper, richer broth, I like to go 8 to 12 hours. Using a ladle, carefully skim off and discard any foam and fat that rises to the top of the broth every 30 minutes or so.

6 Once you reach the depth of flavor you like, remove from the heat and strain, discarding the solids. Return the broth to the pot, season with salt, and add the grated ginger.

7 Drink or use immediately, or store in airtight containers in the refrigerator for up to 1 week or freeze for up to 3 months.

TECHNIQUE TIP: Chef Marco Canora taught me a great trick: Freeze cold stock in glass jars without their lids so the glass doesn't crack. Once frozen, screw on the lids.

This is a vegetarian soup that has lots of deep flavors. I like to make it with Mushroom Broth (page 143), but it can be done just as easily with your favorite stock (pages 138 to 141). I cook a little rice directly into the soup to add some texture and help bring all the vegetables together.

SERVES
4 TO 6

MUSHROOM MISO SOUP WITH DELICATA SQUASH AND GREENS

8 cups Mushroom Broth
(recipe follows)

2 tablespoons gluten-free miso paste

1 tablespoon gluten-free tamari

1 tablespoon rice vinegar

1 cup black rice, soaked overnight

1 delicata squash, scrubbed, halved, seeded, and cut into ½-inch-thick half-moons

2 carrots, cut into 1-inch chunks

1 cup shiitake mushroom caps, stems reserved for broth (recipe follows)

4 leeks, white and pale green parts only, cut into 1-inch-thick rounds

4 garlic cloves, sliced

1 cup kombu seaweed, rinsed and cut into ½-inch strips

2 cups thinly sliced kale leaves

Cilantro sprigs

Lime wedges

1   Bring the broth to a boil in a large saucepot. Whisk in the miso, tamari, and vinegar.

2   Drain the rice, rinse well, and add it to the broth. Adjust the heat to maintain a steady simmer and simmer for 15 minutes.

3   Add the squash, carrots, mushrooms, leeks, garlic, and kombu. Simmer until the rice is tender and the vegetables are just cooked through, 15 to 20 minutes.

4   Add the kale and stir until just wilted. Serve immediately, garnished with the cilantro, and with lime wedges alongside for squeezing.

NOTE: When trimming the shiitake mushrooms, reserve the stems for the Mushroom Broth (recipe follows). Do the same with the green tops of the leeks.

MUSHROOM BROTH MAKES ABOUT 8 CUPS

I created this broth as the base of my Mushroom Miso Soup with Delicata Squash and Greens (page 142) and use the vegetable scraps from that soup to season this broth. But you don't have to make the miso soup to enjoy this broth. Use whatever vegetable scraps you have on hand, then drink the broth as a tea. You can season it with a little gluten-free tamari and a drop of vinegar, if you'd like.

4 cups dried shiitakes, plus any fresh shiitake stems or mushroom scraps (see page 142)

4 pieces dried kombu seaweed, rinsed

4 green leek tops (see page 142)

Jacobsen flake finishing sea salt and freshly ground black pepper

1   In a large stockpot, combine the shiitakes, kombu, leeks, and 12 cups cold water. Bring to a boil, then reduce the heat to maintain a simmer and cook for 1 hour.

2   Strain through a fine-mesh sieve and discard the solids. Season with salt and pepper. Use immediately or transfer to airtight containers and refrigerate for up to 2 weeks or freeze for up to 6 months.

BLACK RICE

It's also known by the brand name Forbidden rice because it used to be forbidden to anyone but the emperor in ancient China. The dark color reflects the high level of antioxidants, which makes it good for your immune system. Its nutty taste and chewiness make it really satisfying, especially after a hard workout. It takes longer to cook than white grains, but it's worth the wait.

I love squash soup so much, I could eat it every day all fall and winter. In fact, I sort of do. If you're making this for yourself, the soup and kefir sauce will keep in the fridge all week. To add a little crunch, sprinkle toasted pepitas on top.

ROASTED WINTER SQUASH SOUP WITH KEFIR AND OLIVE OIL

4 cups 1-inch chunks peeled and seeded butternut or kabocha squash

2 shallots, thinly sliced

4 garlic cloves

2 bay leaves

4 thyme sprigs

1 dried chile

¼ cup champagne vinegar or white wine vinegar

¾ cup extra-virgin olive oil

Jacobsen flake finishing sea salt and freshly ground black pepper

2 cups plain full-fat kefir

6 cups Vegetable Stock (page 138), hot

1 lemon

1 Preheat the oven to 400°F. In a large roasting pan, toss the squash, shallots, garlic, bay leaves, thyme, chile, vinegar, and ¼ cup of the olive oil. Season with salt and pepper. Roast until tender and cooked through, about 35 minutes.

2 Remove and discard the bay leaves, thyme, and chile. In a cup or bowl with a spout, whisk 1 cup of the kefir with ¼ cup of the oil. Transfer everything from the roasting pan to a blender, add the stock, and puree until very smooth. With the blender running, add the kefir mixture in a slow, steady stream. Season with salt and pepper.

3 In a medium bowl, whisk together the remaining 1 cup kefir and the remaining ¼ cup oil. Zest the lemon into the mixture and whisk well. Season with salt and pepper. Divide the soup among serving bowls and drizzle with the kefir sauce.

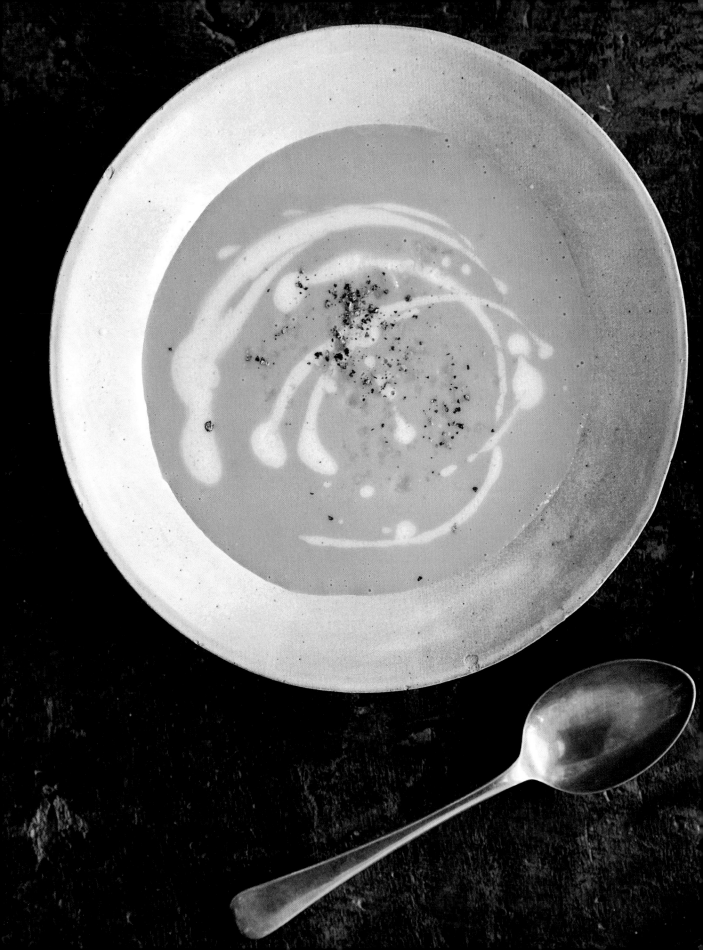

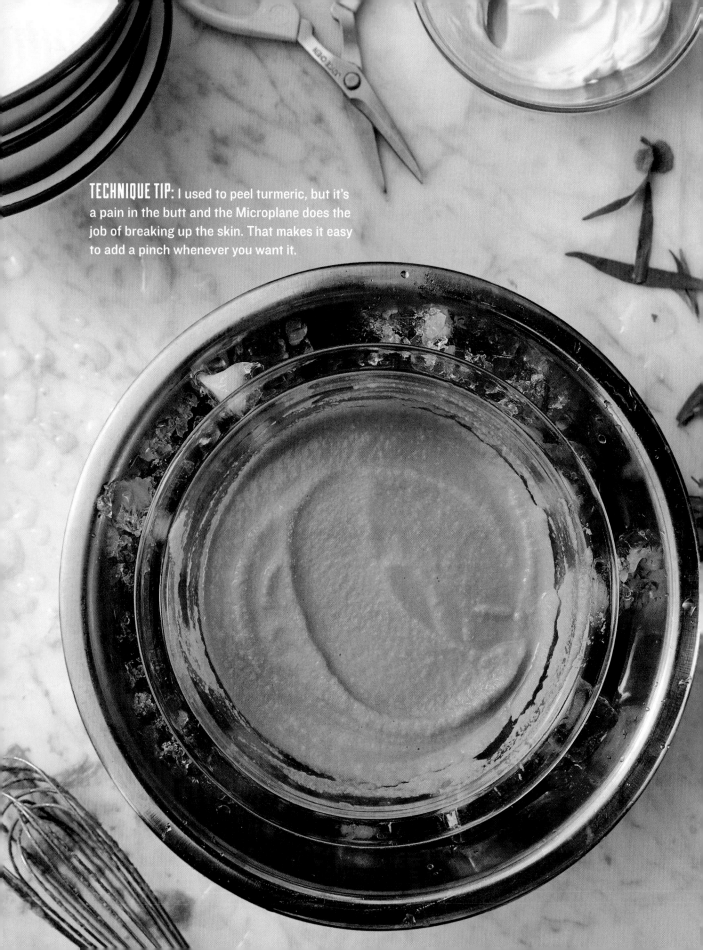

TECHNIQUE TIP: I used to peel turmeric, but it's a pain in the butt and the Microplane does the job of breaking up the skin. That makes it easy to add a pinch whenever you want it.

A cup of this soup will make you feel so good—and keep you from getting sick. Both ginger and turmeric are anti-inflammatory, carrots are loaded with antioxidants, and orange delivers vitamin C. And they all taste amazing together.

SERVES 4 TO 6

CHILLED CARROT SOUP WITH CITRUS AND GINGER

Kosher salt and freshly ground black pepper

I pound large carrots, trimmed and scrubbed

I shallot, diced

I garlic clove, finely diced

I tablespoon raw apple cider vinegar

I tablespoon grated peeled fresh ginger

¼ teaspoon grated fresh turmeric

I orange

½ cup extra-virgin olive oil

Jacobsen flake finishing sea salt

½ cup labne

Fresh tarragon leaves, chopped

Bring a large saucepan of generously salted water to a boil. Fill a large bowl with ice and salted water. Add the carrots to the boiling water and cook until bright orange and crisp-tender, about 5 minutes. Transfer to the ice water. When cool, drain well, chop, and transfer to a blender.

Add the shallot, garlic, vinegar, ginger, and turmeric to the blender. Zest one-quarter of the orange into the blender, then squeeze in all the juice from the orange. Puree on high speed until smooth, adding a little cold water if needed to get the blender going. With the machine running on low speed, add the olive oil in a slow, steady stream. Puree until fully incorporated. Season with sea salt and pepper.

Refrigerate until well chilled. Season again with sea salt and pepper before serving. Divide among bowls and top with the labne and tarragon.

When you taste this, you'll think it could sort of be Vietnamese or Thai or Japanese. It's none of them. I guess I'd call it pseudo-Asian. It's not fusion or a bastardized version of any one cuisine. For example, coconut is never used in Japanese cooking. But when you sip the broth, it makes complete sense. With loads of vegetables and chicken, it's the perfect one-bowl meal.

CHICKEN SOUP WITH GINGER, LEEKS, MUSHROOMS, OKRA, AND BOK CHOY

2 tablespoons coconut oil

3 chicken legs (about 1½ pounds)

Jacobsen flake finishing sea salt and freshly ground black pepper

1 small winter squash, peeled, seeded, and cut into 2-inch chunks (2 cups)

2 small leeks, white and pale green parts only, cut into ¾-inch slices (1 cup)

1 teaspoon fish sauce

1 teaspoon soy sauce

1 tablespoon rice vinegar

2 bok choy, leaves kept whole, stems cut into 1-inch slices

4 cups Chicken Stock (page 139) or store-bought unsalted chicken broth

1 garlic clove, thinly sliced

1 (2-inch) piece fresh ginger, peeled and very thinly sliced

12 okra pods, trimmed and cut into ½-inch slices

10 shiitake mushrooms, stemmed, caps quartered

½ long red chile, seeded, if desired, and thinly sliced

Cilantro

Lime wedges

Heat a large Dutch oven over high heat. Add the coconut oil and swirl to coat the bottom of the pan. Generously season the chicken with salt and pepper and add it to the hot oil, skin-side down. Cook until the skin is golden brown, about 8 minutes. Flip the legs over and reduce the heat to medium-low.

Add the squash and cook, stirring occasionally, until lightly browned, about 6 minutes. Add the leeks and fish sauce and stir well. Add the soy sauce, stir, then add the vinegar and stir again. Let the liquids bubble and reduce a bit.

RECIPE CONTINUES ▶

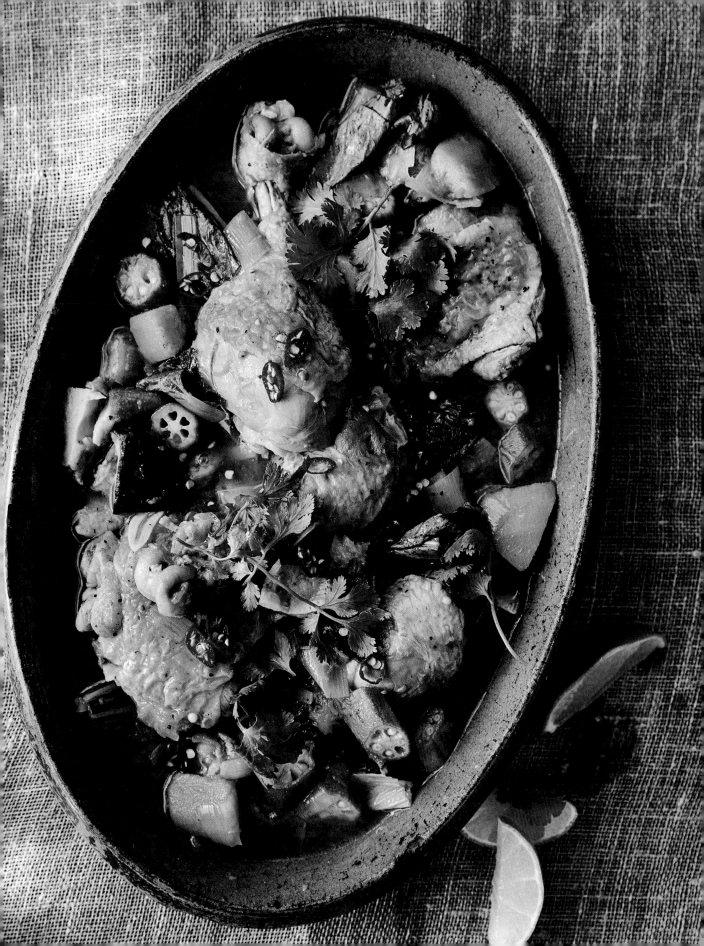

3 Add the bok choy stems and stock and bring to a boil. Reduce the heat to low and season with salt. Add the garlic and ginger and simmer for a minute, then add the okra and mushrooms. Simmer until the okra is just cooked through, about 6 minutes.

4 Season with salt and pepper, then stir in the chile. Add the bok choy greens and fold in just until wilted, about 1 minute. Divide among serving bowls and top with cilantro. Serve immediately, with the lime wedges alongside.

TECHNIQUE TIP: I'm amazed when people throw everything in the pot at the same time for soup. They miss the beautiful alchemy of cooking. When I make broth-based soups, I add the vegetables in the order of how long they need to cook. The things that take longest to soften should go in first and then wind down until everything is cooked the right amount. For example, you'd go from carrots to squash to onion to garlic to tomato to spinach. I never want anything to end up mushy, and I prefer leaves just wilted.

Cold and creamy, sweet and tangy, this is the ultimate late-summer soup. It's so refreshing, but it tastes rich with olive oil blended in. A big bowl for lunch is all I need on a hot day.

CUCUMBER AND HONEYDEW GAZPACHO

¼ cup champagne vinegar

2 garlic cloves

Jacobsen flake finishing sea salt and freshly ground black pepper

3 very large regular cucumbers, peeled, seeded, and diced (about 4 cups)

1 large honeydew, peeled, seeded, and cut into chunks (about 4 cups)

¾ cup extra-virgin olive oil, plus more for serving

1 lemon

Fresh basil leaves

Espelette pepper

1 Put the vinegar in a blender. Grate the garlic directly into the vinegar with a Microplane and add 2 teaspoons salt. Let sit for a few minutes, then add the cucumbers and honeydew. Blend on high speed until very smooth, adding a bit of water if needed to get the blender going. Work in batches, if necessary.

2 With the machine running, add the olive oil through the feed tube in a slow, steady stream. When it's completely emulsified, season with salt and pepper. Zest the lemon directly into the mixture and whisk in until fully incorporated. Refrigerate until very cold.

3 Before serving, stir or blend until smooth again. Divide among serving bowls and drizzle with olive oil. Tear the basil leaves and scatter them on top, and sprinkle with Espelette. Serve immediately.

On hot, humid summer days, I crave refreshing midday meals that won't leave me feeling gross. My spin on Spanish gazpacho hits the spot. I keep a pitcher in the fridge and pour myself a glass whenever a craving strikes. The base recipe below fills me up, but you can top it with wild crabmeat for a more substantial meal.

MAKES 8 CUPS;
SERVES 4 TO 8

TOMATO AND WATERMELON GAZPACHO

4 cups diced vine-ripened tomatoes

4 cups diced seedless watermelon, plus finely diced watermelon for serving

I cup diced red bell pepper

I cup diced peeled and seeded English cucumber

I garlic clove, smashed

¼ cup sherry vinegar

½ cup extra-virgin olive oil, plus more for serving

Jacobsen flake finishing sea salt and freshly ground black pepper

Diced avocado

Fresh basil, torn

In a blender, combine the tomatoes, watermelon, bell pepper, cucumber, garlic, and vinegar. (If your blender jar isn't large enough to hold the ingredients, put them in a bowl.) Cover and refrigerate overnight.

When ready to serve, blend until smooth, working in batches, if necessary. With the machine running, add the olive oil in a slow, steady stream. Season with salt and pepper.

Divide among serving glasses and top with avocado, basil, and finely diced watermelon. Drizzle with olive oil and serve immediately.

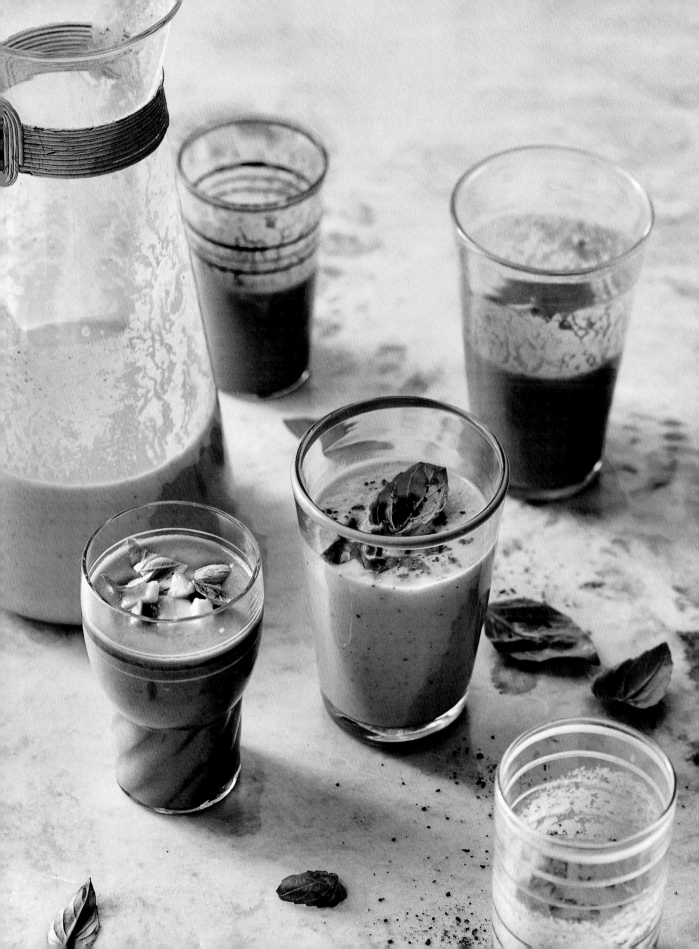

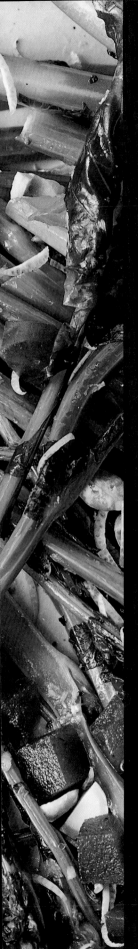

BLANCHING AND SHOCKING VEGETABLES

One thing we chefs learn early on in our first kitchen apprenticeships is the value of blanching and shocking vegetables.

- **Blanching Vegetables:** Blanching is simply cooking vegetables in a large pot of well-salted boiling water until they're 70 percent done. Make sure the water is as salty as the sea, and I mean the Dead Sea! It's really important to blanch your veggies in small batches and to allow the water to come back up to a rapid boil after each batch. If the water isn't at a strong rolling boil, you won't be able to quickly cook and "set" the veggies.

- **Shocking Vegetables:** The second part of the trick is stopping the cooking. Even after you turn off the stove, there will be carryover cooking, which means residual heat will continue to cook the vegetables. And simply running cold water over the vegetables won't cool them down quickly enough. So what to do? Drain the vegetables fast and immediately plunge them into an ice water bath. The proper ratio for a successful ice water bath is 2 parts ice to 3 parts cold water.

- **How to Do It Fast:** To make blanching and shocking efficient, I start by bringing my big pot of salted water to a boil. While that's heating up, I prep my vegetables. Then I prepare a large ice water bath. After the vegetables have cooked and cooled completely, I drain them again and pat them dry. I can then cook them right away, or set them aside in the fridge for later.

- **Why Do It:** You now have a stash of vegetables ready for a quick breakfast, lunch, or dinner. The other reason is technical: Blanching and shocking allow you to perfectly cook every ingredient when putting together a dish. Have you ever sautéed some eggplant, asparagus, and broccoli rabe together and found that by the time the eggplant is cooked through, the asparagus looks drab? Is it a sad army green rather than bright and vibrant? Well, you've actually lost a lot of the nutrients and flavor along with the color. If you blanch and shock vegetables and then sauté them, you can make sure everything comes out cooked to perfection! Much healthier and much, much tastier.

Blending sugar snaps with shell peas keeps the texture of my spring soup less starchy than the standard. If you want to highlight the sweetness of the peas, you can substitute white balsamic vinegar for the sherry vinegar.

CHILLED PEA SOUP WITH YOGURT

Kosher salt

8 ounces sugar snap peas

8 ounces shelled English peas or thawed frozen peas

½ cup plus I tablespoon extra-virgin olive oil

2 shallots, minced

I garlic clove, minced

I tablespoon fino sherry vinegar

5 cups Vegetable Stock (page 138) or store-bought unsalted vegetable broth

I cup plain full-fat yogurt

Zest and juice of I lemon

I cup loosely packed fresh mint leaves

Sea salt and freshly ground black pepper

Herbed Yogurt (page 290)

Bring a large pot of generously salted water to a boil. Fill a large bowl with salted water and ice. Add snap peas to the boiling water and cook until bright green, about 1 minute. Transfer to the ice water with a slotted spoon. Bring the water in the pot back to a boil. Add the peas and cook until bright green, about 1 minute for frozen and 2 to 3 minutes for fresh. Drain and transfer to the ice water. When cool, drain all the peas well.

In a large saucepan, heat 1 tablespoon of the olive oil over medium-low heat. Add the shallots and garlic and cook, stirring, until translucent, about 2 minutes. Add the vinegar and cook, stirring, until reduced completely. Remove from the heat.

In a blender, combine the snap peas, peas, shallot mixture, and stock and puree on high speed until smooth. Add the plain yogurt, scraping the bowl, and puree until smooth. With the machine running on low speed, add the remaining ½ cup oil in a slow, steady stream. Puree until fully incorporated. Add the lemon zest, lemon juice, and mint and puree until smooth. Season with sea salt and pepper. Refrigerate until well chilled. Season again with salt and pepper before serving. Divide among bowls and top with the herbed yogurt.

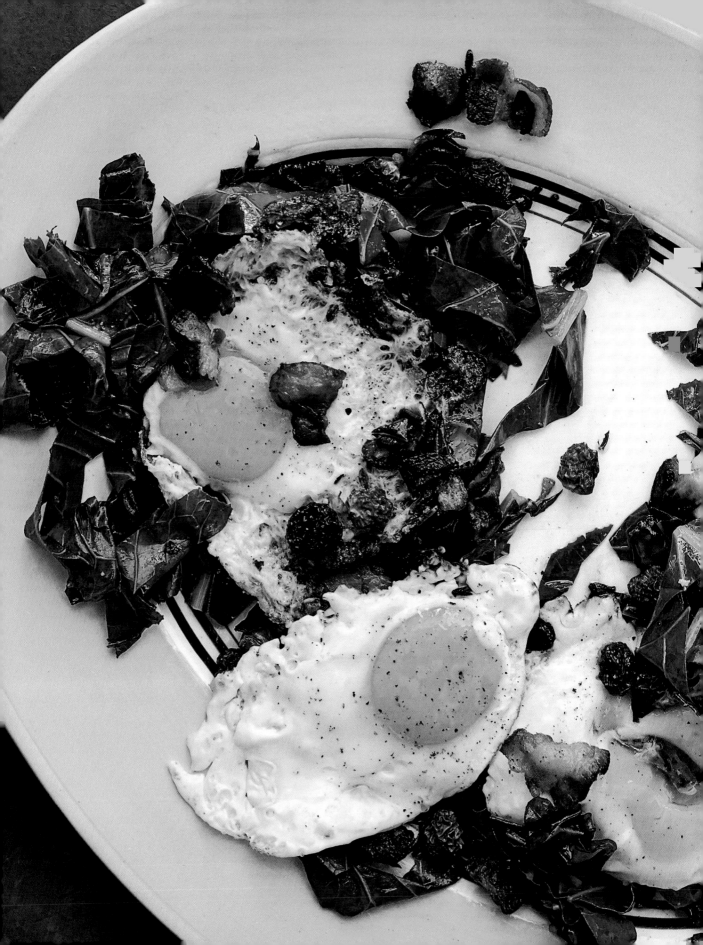

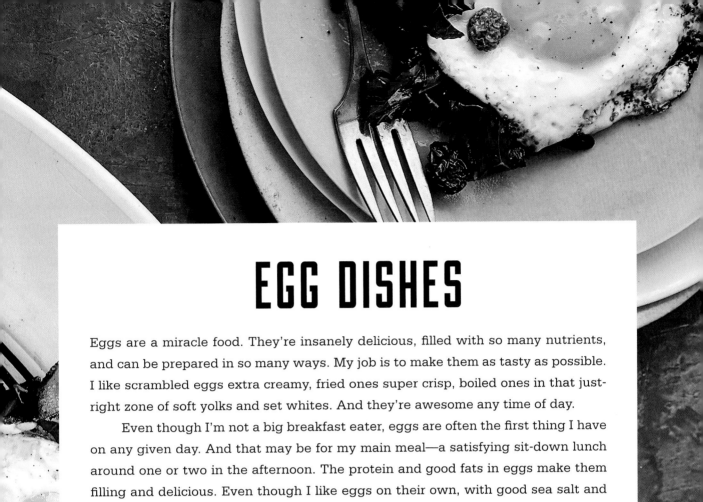

EGG DISHES

Eggs are a miracle food. They're insanely delicious, filled with so many nutrients, and can be prepared in so many ways. My job is to make them as tasty as possible. I like scrambled eggs extra creamy, fried ones super crisp, boiled ones in that just-right zone of soft yolks and set whites. And they're awesome any time of day.

Even though I'm not a big breakfast eater, eggs are often the first thing I have on any given day. And that may be for my main meal—a satisfying sit-down lunch around one or two in the afternoon. The protein and good fats in eggs make them filling and delicious. Even though I like eggs on their own, with good sea salt and freshly ground black pepper, I really enjoy them over other dishes, too. I'll often slide a fried egg over roasted vegetables, a hearty salad, or even a lamb patty. Breaking the runny yolks and slashing them into any dish creates an instant and crazy good sauce.

Be sure to buy pastured eggs or organic eggs, preferably from a local farmer. The official "organic" label ensures that the chickens are cage-free and given organic feed. Vendors at your farmers' market may have smaller operations that can't afford to get that designation, but they may very well be organic and they'll definitely be fresher.

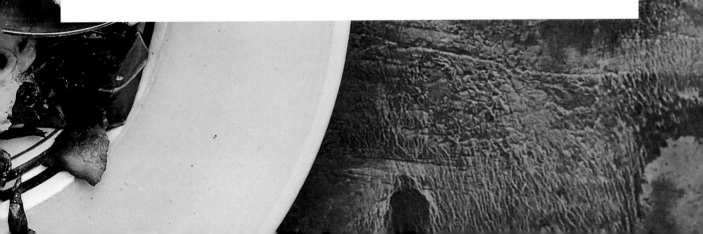

Most mornings, I'm not hungry enough to eat breakfast right when I get up. After a long stretch of events and traveling, though, I sometimes wake up really hungry and really tired. On those mornings, I'll make myself this full plate—and lots of coffee. To get the most out of this meal, I break the yolks to let them run all over, then try to get a bit of everything with each bite. If I'm really hungry, I'll have a slice of gluten-free Le Pain Quotidien toast with grass-fed butter, too.

SERVES 1

BACON AND EGGS WITH KIMCHI

¾ ounce slab bacon, cut into slices

Avocado oil

2 large eggs

Kimchi

1 In a large cast-iron skillet, cook the bacon over medium heat, turning occasionally, until the fat renders and the bacon is dark golden brown, about 6 minutes.

2 At the same time, in a large cast-iron skillet, heat a thin layer of avocado oil over high heat until very hot. Add the eggs and cook until the whites are just set and the yolks are runny.

3 Slide the eggs and bacon onto a serving plate and mound the kimchi on the side. Cut it all up and eat everything together.

HEALTH TIP: Yes, I do occasionally have a slice of gluten-free toast. But it's not because I think that will cure me. We have this causality notion about health. If we can figure out the cause, then we can find a solution. But our bodies are more complex than that. There are a multitude of circumstances that lead to poor health—and just as many that can fix it. So you can't simply say, "I'm allergic to gluten and I'm going to cut it out and find a gluten-free bread I like." You have to look at the whole spectrum of what you're eating and see how everything adds up. Microchanges across the whole spectrum of your diet will lead to macro results.

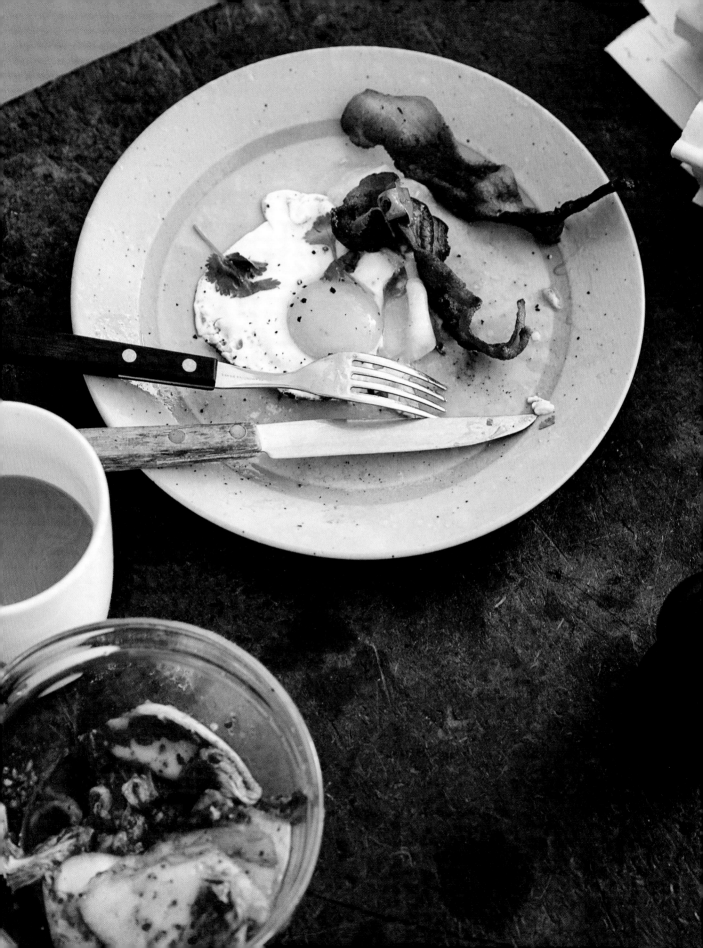

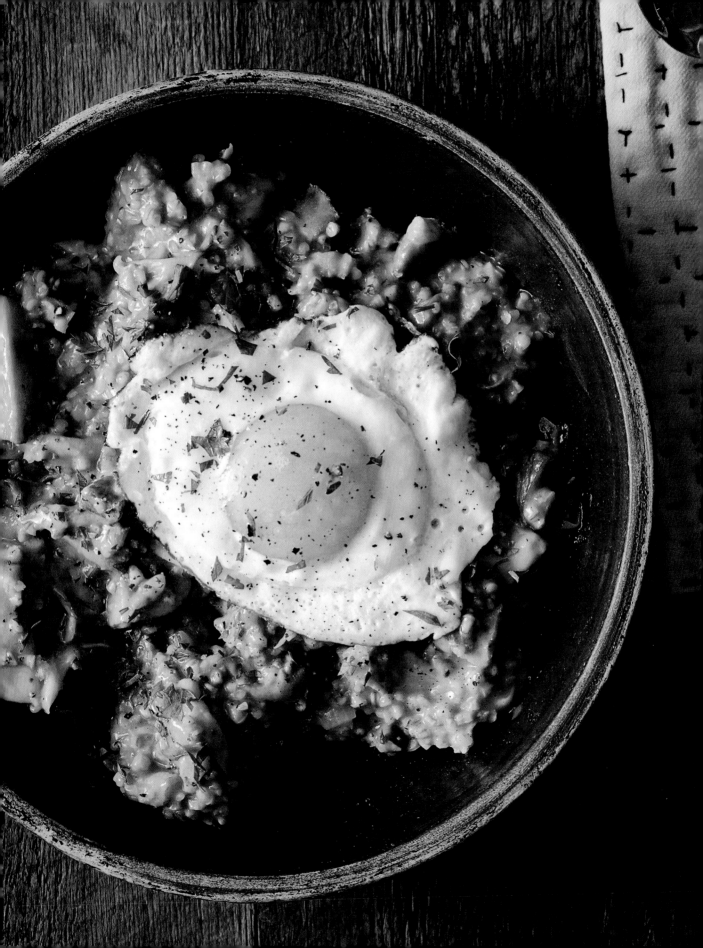

Stirring oats as they simmer in stock yields a dish with the creaminess of risotto. But steel-cut oats have an added depth, especially when they're cooked with bacon and wild mushrooms. This dish is especially good if made with Irish grass-fed butter and cheese.

SAVORY OATS WITH BACON, MUSHROOMS, AND FRIED EGGS

I teaspoon extra-virgin olive oil

½ cup diced double-smoked bacon

I shallot, finely diced

8 ounces mixed fresh wild mushrooms

I teaspoon white wine vinegar

2 cups Irish steel-cut oats

4 cups Chicken Stock (page 139) or store-bought unsalted chicken broth, heated

½ cup finely grated cheddar cheese

2 tablespoons grass-fed unsalted butter

Jacobsen flake finishing sea salt and freshly ground black pepper

4 fried eggs (see page 162)

2 tablespoons coarsely chopped fresh flat-leaf parsley

1   In a large, heavy saucepan, heat the olive oil over medium heat. Add the bacon and cook, stirring often, until golden brown, about 8 minutes.

2   Add the shallot and mushrooms and cook, stirring often, until the shallot is translucent, about 2 minutes. Add the vinegar and cook, stirring and scraping, until the mushrooms are moist but there's a little liquid in the bottom of the pan, 2 to 3 minutes.

3   Toss in the oats, then add a ladleful of the chicken stock and stir with a silicone spatula. As the oats absorb the liquid, continuously add a bit more just as you would to make a risotto, stirring the whole time. All the liquid should have been added and the oats fully cooked through after about 15 minutes.

4   Add the cheese and butter and gently fold until thoroughly incorporated. Season with salt and pepper. Divide the oats among four serving dishes and top each with a fried egg. Sprinkle with parsley and serve.

Straight-up bacon strips taste best crunchy, but here, I don't want diced slab bacon to end up crisp. I like the saltiness of the toothsome cubes against the sweetness of chewy dried berries, all tangled up in greens. Fried eggs on top are amazing for breakfast or brunch—or even dinner—but you can serve just the greens as a small plate, too.

FRIED EGGS OVER BACON, GOLDEN BERRY, AND COLLARDS SAUTÉ

1½ ounces slab bacon, cut into ½-inch batons

I small bunch collard greens, tough ribs removed, cut into ½-inch slices

I shallot, halved and thinly sliced

I garlic clove, very thinly sliced

3 tablespoons dried golden berries (page 105) or dried sour cherries

FRIED EGGS

Avocado oil or extra-virgin olive oil, for frying

4 large eggs, at room temperature

Jacobsen flake finishing sea salt and freshly ground black pepper

1 In a large cast-iron skillet, cook the bacon over medium heat, stirring occasionally, until the fat renders, about 5 minutes. Add the collards and cook, stirring, for 1 minute. Add the shallot and garlic and cook, stirring, just until the greens wilt, about 1 minute. Stir in the berries.

2 To make the fried eggs, in a large cast-iron skillet, heat a thin layer of avocado oil over high heat until very hot. Add the eggs and cook until the whites are just set and the yolks are runny. Season with salt and pepper.

3 Serve the eggs over the greens.

TECHNIQUE TIP: Adding aromatics like shallot and garlic to greens after they wilt prevents them from burning. Instead, they gently weep into the greens.

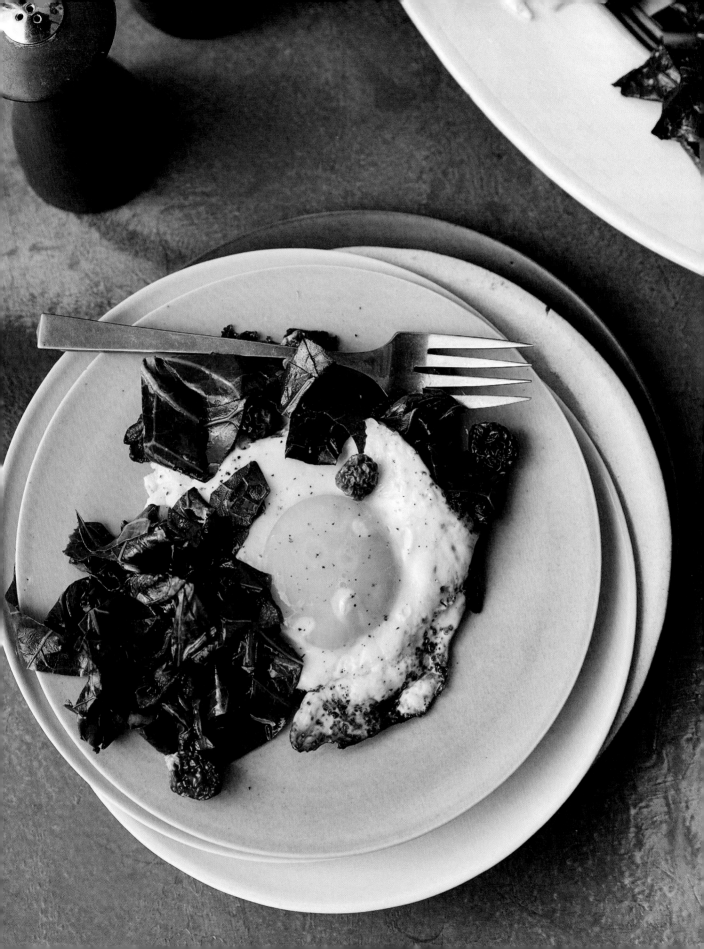

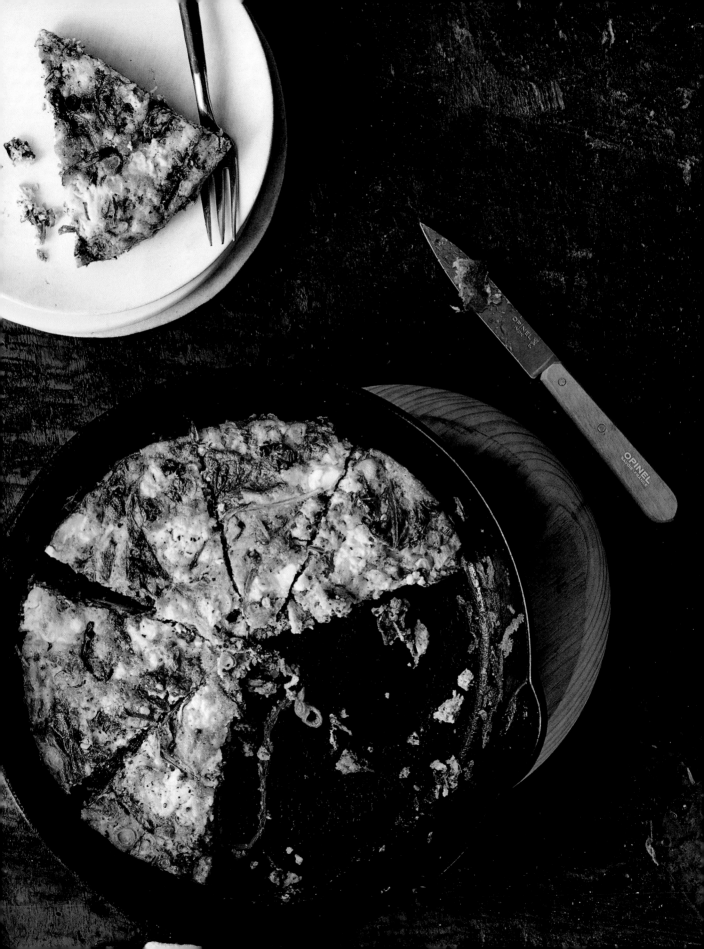

This is a perfect brunch dish because it's really rich and flavorful. So much so that it even tastes good cold, so you can make it ahead of time. The combination of lamb and eggs is common in lots of other cultures, including Middle Eastern ones, which inspired my use of za'atar spice. I use a blend that's already mixed with olive oil. If you buy the spice dry, mix 1 tablespoon za'atar with 1 tablespoon olive oil to create a paste.

SERVES
4 TO 6

KALE, LAMB, AND FETA FRITTATA

4 ounces ground lamb (77% lean)

2 tablespoons za'atar spice blend with olive oil (see headnote)

Jacobsen flake finishing sea salt and freshly ground black pepper

8 large eggs

2 tablespoons plain full-fat yogurt

3 tablespoons fresh cilantro

2 tablespoons fresh tarragon leaves

1 tablespoon fresh basil leaves

2 spring onions or scallions, very thinly sliced

2 cups baby kale

¼ cup crumbled feta cheese

1 tablespoon extra-virgin olive oil

1 Preheat the oven to 425°F.

2 In a medium bowl, combine the lamb, za'atar, and 1 teaspoon salt and mix until the lamb is evenly seasoned.

3 Break the eggs into a large bowl and whisk until the eggs are broken. Add the yogurt and season with salt and pepper. Whisk again until smooth. Tear in the cilantro, tarragon, and basil, then add the spring onions, kale, and feta. Stir well.

RECIPE CONTINUES ▶

FETA CHEESE

All salty feta cheese is really good, but I much prefer the kind made with sheep's milk because of its funky flavor.

4 Heat a 9- to 10-inch cast-iron skillet over high heat. Add the olive oil and swirl to coat the bottom of the pan. When the oil is hot, add the lamb mixture. Cook, stirring and breaking the meat up into little bits, until the lamb is browned, about 2 minutes.

5 Add the egg mixture and stir once or twice. Use a silicone spatula to spread out the egg and tuck in the set egg around the edges of the pan. Poke the meat and vegetables around until they're evenly distributed. Transfer the pan to the oven.

6 Bake until the egg is just set, 7 to 10 minutes. Loosen the edges of the egg with a spatula.

7 Serve the frittata hot, warm, or room temperature straight out of the pan, cutting it into wedges.

SECRETS TO THE BEST SCRAMBLED EGGS

- Start with a well-seasoned cast-iron pan. It's more nonstick than nonstick.

- Use a silicone spatula to stir, not a wooden or metal spoon, because its soft edges allow you to scrape the pans well.

- Stirring chia seeds into the beaten eggs adds pop and crunch to the finished plate of soft, creamy eggs. Plus, they're rich in good fats.

- Mixing cold butter bits into the beaten eggs allows the butter to emulsify with the egg proteins as they cook, making the scramble even creamier.

- Eat them hot and unadorned or throw in avocados after scrambling for more creaminess and good fats. Fold in your favorite soft herbs for a fresh hit.

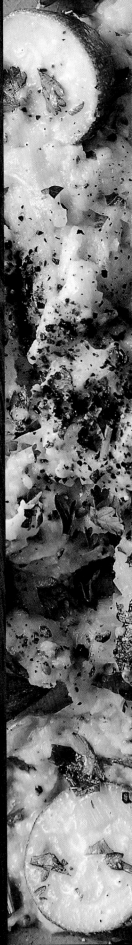

Even though this dish can come together quickly on a weekday morning, it's perfect for a leisurely weekend brunch. Chia seeds give the eggs an especially creamy texture, as does just a bit of grass-fed butter. The combination of avocado and salmon makes this satisfying enough to hold you over until dinner—or to make it a nice dinner.

SERVES 2 TO 4

SOFT SCRAMBLED EGGS WITH AVOCADO, CHIA SEEDS, SMOKED SALMON, AND KALE

5 large eggs

2 tablespoons unsalted grass-fed butter, cut into small pieces

1 tablespoon chopped fresh dill

1 teaspoon chia seeds

2 ounces smoked wild salmon, thinly sliced

1 tablespoon extra-virgin olive oil

4 Tuscan kale leaves, thinly sliced

1 garlic clove, thinly sliced

1 avocado, pitted, peeled, and cut into ½-inch pieces

Jacobsen flake finishing sea salt and freshly ground black pepper

1 Lightly beat the eggs in a medium bowl. Fold in the butter, dill, chia seeds, and smoked salmon.

2 In a medium well-seasoned cast-iron or nonstick skillet, heat the olive oil over medium-low heat. Add the kale and cook, stirring, to gently wilt, about 1 minute. Add the garlic and stir for another minute, then add the egg mixture. With a silicone spatula, gently fold the egg mixture until creamy and lightly scrambled but still a little moist. Fold in the avocado at the very last minute, season with salt and pepper, and serve right away.

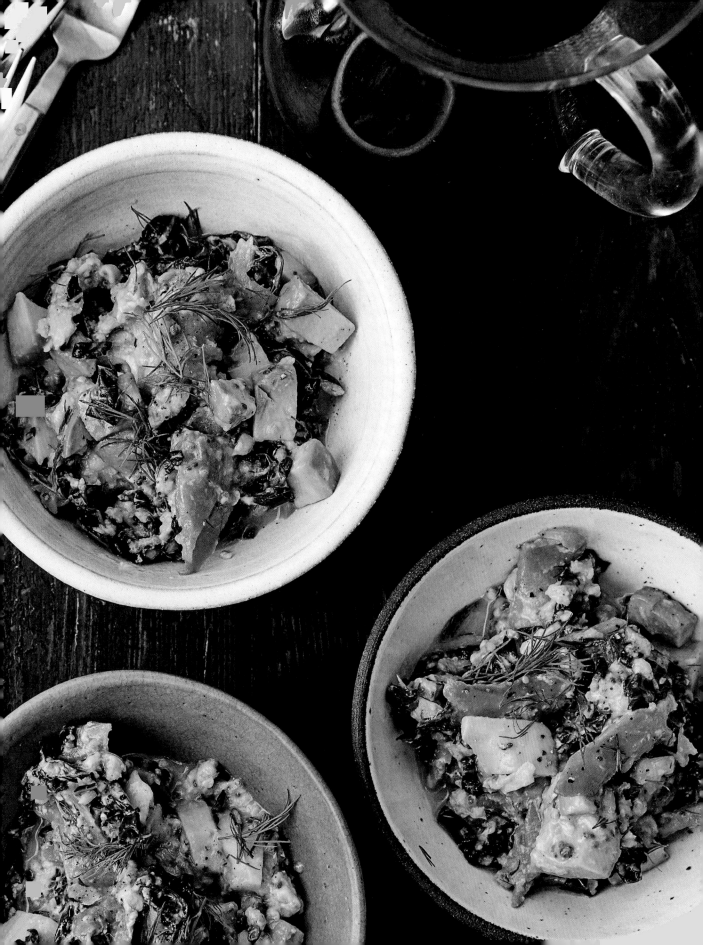

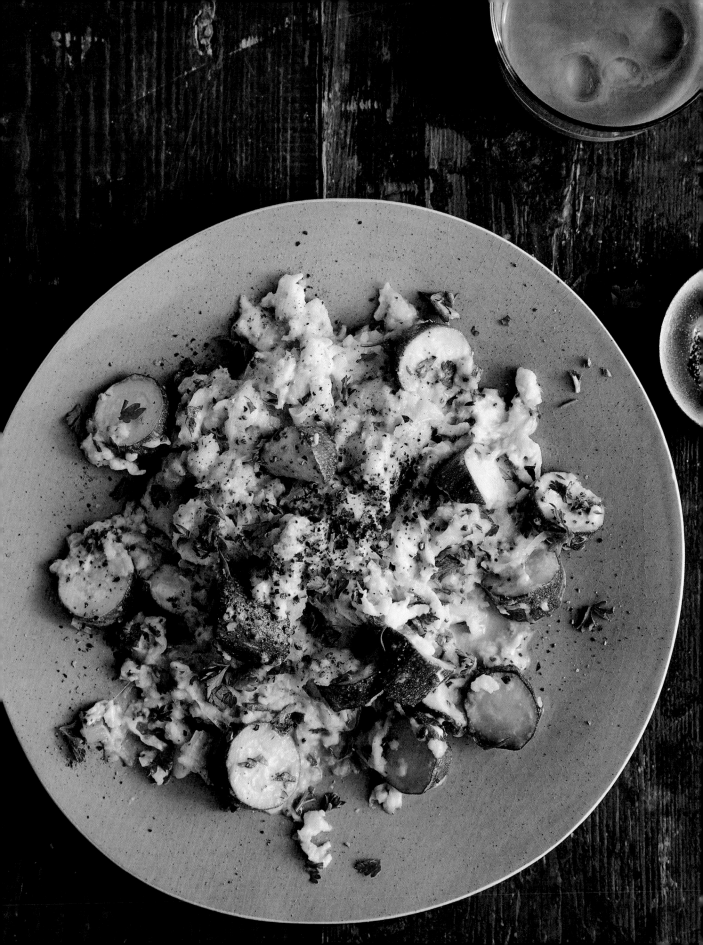

I really love the way summer squash tastes when it's just wilted. To get that nice, crunchy texture, I avoid cutting it into thin slices. Seedy slices weep, making the eggs watery. Instead, I cut a halved squash into larger chunks. That reduces the moisture it releases and keeps the squash crisp when nestled in the creamy eggs.

SCRAMBLED EGGS WITH LEEKS, SQUASH, AND HERBS

6 large eggs

Jacobsen flake finishing sea salt and freshly ground black pepper

2 teaspoons chia seeds

4 tablespoons grass-fed unsalted butter, cut into small pieces

¼ cup thinly sliced leeks (white and pale green parts only)

1 small summer squash, such as zucchini, halved lengthwise and cut into ¾-inch chunks at angles

¼ teaspoon champagne vinegar

¼ cup fresh curly parsley, chopped

¼ cup fresh cilantro, chopped

Espelette pepper or pimentón (smoked sweet paprika)

1 Beat the eggs in a large bowl with a fork until a little bubbly but still retaining some white streaks. Season with salt and black pepper, then fold in the chia seeds and 2 tablespoons of the butter. Let stand so the chia seeds can plump while you prepare the vegetables.

2 Heat a large cast-iron skillet over medium-low heat. Add the remaining 2 tablespoons butter, the leeks, and the squash. Season with salt and cook, stirring occasionally, for 1 minute. Add the vinegar and let it cook off, then add the egg mixture.

3 Use a silicone spatula to stir and scrape the set eggs around the edges of the pan into the wet center, then let them sit for a minute. They should start to set. Add the parsley and cilantro and fold well until the eggs are moist but not runny, 1 to 2 minutes.

4 Remove from the heat and sprinkle with Espelette. Serve immediately.

This is a healthy, balanced breakfast of good fats, proteins, and vegetables. Even though this omelet is done in two steps, it takes ten minutes at most. It's especially good with Fra Mani smoked ham, which is nitrate-free and made with pastured, naturally raised pork.

MUSHROOM, ASPARAGUS, AND HAM OMELET

3 large eggs

Jacobsen flake finishing sea salt and freshly ground black pepper

1 tablespoon grass-fed unsalted butter

1 cup mixed fresh mushrooms, coarsely chopped

3 asparagus stalks, trimmed and cut into 3-inch pieces

2 slices highest-quality ham, cut into strips

¼ cup finely grated aged cheddar cheese (optional)

2 fresh basil leaves, chopped

1   In a medium bowl, lightly beat the eggs with a pinch each of salt and pepper.

2   In a medium cast-iron skillet, melt the butter over medium-high heat. Once the butter begins to foam, add the mushrooms and cook, stirring, for 1 minute. Add the asparagus and ham and cook, stirring, until the asparagus turns bright green, about 1 minute.

3   Add the eggs and use a silicone spatula to carefully fold in the edges of the omelet while tilting the pan with your other hand so the eggs can run from the center to fill in the whole surface of the pan. Once the eggs are nearly all cooked, sprinkle with the cheese (if using). Add the basil, then slide the omelet out of the pan onto a plate, folding it into a half-moon shape. Serve immediately.

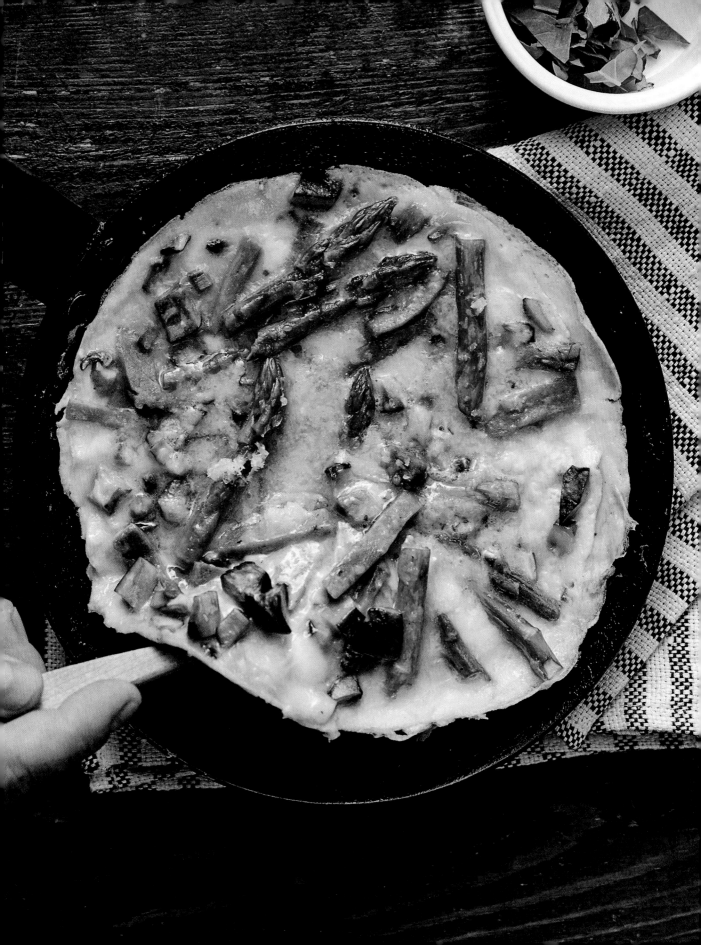

When winter is finally over, I really get excited about spring vegetables, especially wild ones like ramps and fiddlehead ferns. Both are super nutrient-dense and have a ton of flavor—ramps in a spicy sort of garlicky way and fiddleheads in a wild forest bitterness. Be sure to save the ramp greens for pesto (see page 294).

This is a delicious dish that can be riffed on in endless ways. Feel free to improvise and leave out the pancetta if that's not your thing. The idea is simply to play around with whatever shows up at the farmers' market.

SERVES 4

POACHED EGGS WITH SPRING VEGETABLES

¼ cup diced pancetta or bacon

1 cup fiddlehead ferns, rinsed

1 small bunch ramps, bulbs only, trimmed (greens reserved for pesto)

1 cup sliced shiitake mushroom caps

1 tablespoon grass-fed unsalted butter

1 garlic clove, sliced

Jacobsen flake finishing sea salt and freshly ground black pepper

1 tablespoon plus 1 teaspoon champagne vinegar

1 cup dandelion greens, coarsely chopped

Minced fresh herbs, such as basil, chives, and tarragon

4 large eggs, cold

Ramp and Almond Pesto (page 294)

4 thin slices high-quality ham

1 In a medium skillet, cook the pancetta over medium heat, stirring often, until browned and crisp, about 5 minutes. Toss in the fiddleheads, ramp bulbs, mushrooms, and butter. Cook, stirring, until the vegetables are just tender, about 4 minutes.

2 Add the garlic, season with salt and pepper, and stir well. Add 1 tablespoon of the vinegar and cook, stirring, until the vegetables are glazed. Toss in the greens and herbs and remove from the heat.

3 Fill a large, wide saucepan with water to a depth of 1½ inches. Bring to a boil over medium heat. Stir in the remaining 1 teaspoon vinegar. Crack an egg into a small dish, then slide it into the simmering water. Quickly repeat with the remaining eggs, then reduce the heat to low to maintain a bare simmer. Poach until the whites are set but the yolks are still runny, 2 to 3 minutes. Remove from the water with a slotted spoon and drain on paper towels.

4 Smear the pesto in four serving dishes. Divide the vegetables among the dishes and slide a poached egg and a slice of ham on top of each. Serve immediately.

RAMPS

Available only in early spring, ramps grow in the wild and must be foraged. Though they're sometimes called wild leeks or onions, they're neither. They look like scallions with pink ends and broad leaves and have a garlicky sharpness that makes them almost tangy. I love their punchy yet nuanced flavor and their stores of vitamins C and A.

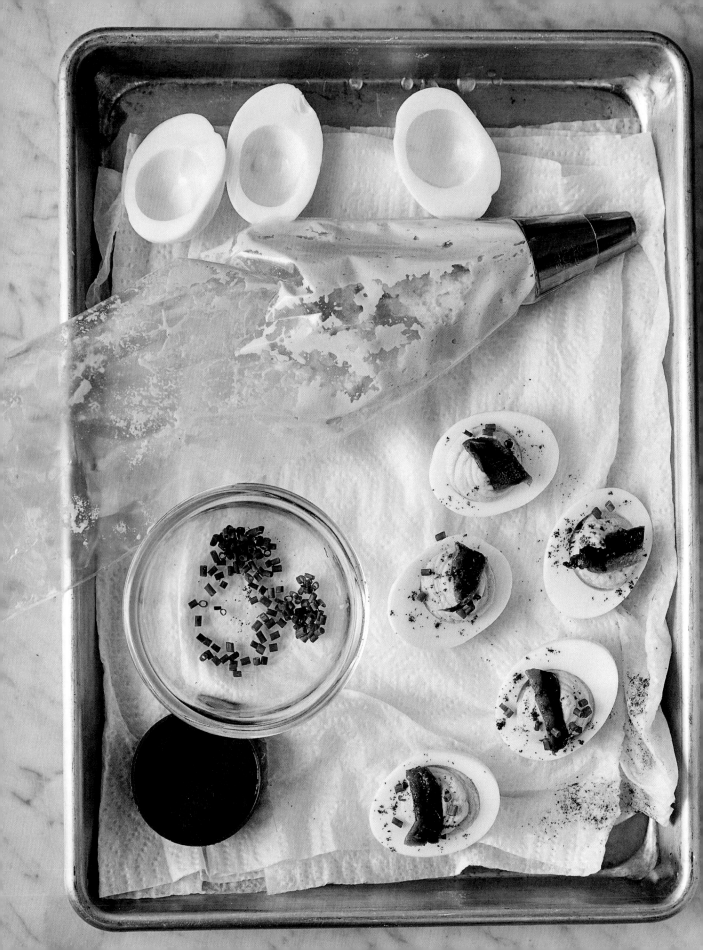

These easy eggs are loaded with antioxidants and healthy fats. And they may just be the most delicious deviled eggs you'll ever have. Anchovies make the creamy filling nice and salty and the rosemary adds a rich herbaceousness.

DEVILED EGGS WITH ANCHOVIES AND ROSEMARY

12 large eggs

3 tablespoons crème fraîche, plus more if needed

1 tablespoon Dijon mustard

¼ teaspoon cayenne pepper

¼ cup extra-virgin olive oil

Juice of ½ lemon

¼ cup fresh rosemary leaves

Jacobsen flake finishing sea salt

12 anchovy fillets, each cut in half

Minced fresh chives

Paprika

1   Bring a large pot of water to a boil. Fill a large bowl with ice and water. Add the eggs to the boiling water and cook for 8 minutes. Drain the eggs and transfer to the ice water. When cool, peel and cut each egg in half lengthwise. Transfer the yolks to the bowl of a food processor; refrigerate the whites.

2   Add the crème fraîche, mustard, cayenne, olive oil, lemon juice, rosemary, and a pinch of salt to the food processor. Process until smooth, scraping the bowl occasionally. The mixture should be soft enough to pipe through a piping bag, but not too loose. If it's stiff, pulse in another tablespoon of crème fraîche. Transfer the mixture to a piping bag or resealable plastic bag with a hole snipped in one corner.

3   Arrange the egg whites cut-side up in a single layer on a serving platter. Pipe the yolk mixture into the egg white cavities. Top each with an anchovy half. Sprinkle with chives and paprika and serve immediately, or refrigerate for up to 2 days.

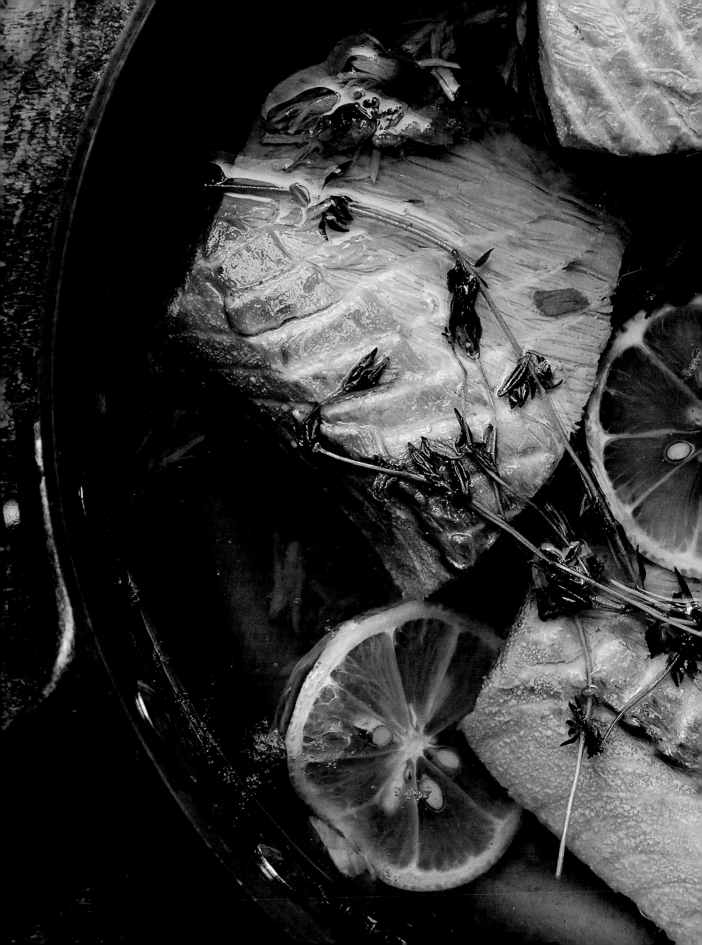

FISH & SEAFOOD

Seafood may be my favorite protein source. It's tasty, takes so well to different seasonings and vegetables, and cooks quickly. The hardest part of preparing seafood is buying it. When creating recipes for this book, I decided to shop at a grocery store instead of getting fish from my restaurant wholesaler to see what you can buy. And it's not pretty. I get that. The flesh may be dry or gaping, the fillets cut in ragged, uneven portions. That's why I've given you foolproof techniques and bold flavors to make sure every dish comes out well.

When looking for seafood, follow these guidelines:

- Buy sustainable fish. A number of watchdog groups, such as the Seafood Watch of the Monterey Bay Aquarium and the Good Fish Guide of the Marine Conservation Society, provide different designations that actually change over time, depending on whether or how fish are being overfished. Wild is generally best, but there are some really great sustainable farming operations, too.

- Seafood shouldn't smell fishy. If you get a whiff of the docks, pass. Good, fresh seafood should smell almost sweet.

- Be flexible. Don't set your heart on one particular type of fish. Instead, choose whichever is freshest or looks best. Fish is fresh when its flesh is gleaming, not dry. It shouldn't gape, either.

- Cook it shortly after you get home. Don't let it sit around for a day.

- The freezer is your friend. Frozen is sometimes your best option. Some sustainable providers individually quick-freeze their catch on the boat, trapping its freshness. That gives you the flexibility to cook fish whenever you want, because it thaws pretty quickly.

For summer dinners, I prefer meals that cook quickly but pack a lot of flavor. Both the salmon and accompanying tomato sauce spend only a little time on the stove, but end up loaded with flavor from rich olive oil. If you happen to have Sauce Vierge (page 299) in the fridge, dollop a teaspoon on each salmon portion for an even bigger savory punch.

SERVES 4

OLIVE OIL-POACHED SALMON WITH TOMATOES AND OLIVES

1 ripe tomato, halved

2 cups plus 2 tablespoons extra-virgin olive oil, plus more for serving

1 lemon, thinly sliced

1 lemon thyme sprig plus 1 tablespoon leaves

4 (3-ounce) pieces skinless wild salmon

Sea salt and freshly ground black pepper

Zest of 1 lemon

2 cups mixed cherry tomatoes

2 shallots, quartered

1 small summer or pattypan squash, cut into ½-inch pieces

1 garlic clove, minced

6 saffron threads

2 tablespoons fino sherry vinegar or white balsamic vinegar

1 tablespoon Niçoise olives, pitted and halved

6 basil leaves, plus more for serving

1   Grate the cut sides of the tomato on the large holes of a box grater set over a bowl to gather the pulp. Discard the skins; set the pulp aside.

2   In a deep skillet, heat 2 cups of the olive oil, the lemon slices, and thyme sprig over low heat until the oil registers 140°F on a deep-fry thermometer. Meanwhile, sprinkle the salmon with salt and pepper. Slide the salmon into the oil, adjusting the heat to maintain the oil temperature. Poach until the fish is just cooked through, 5 to 7 minutes. Carefully transfer to paper towel–lined plates to drain.

3 While the salmon poaches, in a medium saucepan, heat the remaining 2 tablespoons oil over low heat. Add the lemon zest, cherry tomatoes, shallots, and squash. Cook, stirring occasionally, until soft. Stir in the garlic and saffron, then add the vinegar. Cook, stirring, until the vinegar evaporates. Add the grated tomato and simmer until the tomatoes are soft but not cooked down, about 2 minutes. Stir in the olives, basil, and thyme leaves. Season with salt and pepper.

4 Divide the tomato mixture among serving dishes and top with the salmon. Sprinkle more basil leaves on top and drizzle with oil. Serve immediately.

TIP: Strain the poaching oil through a fine-mesh sieve; it can be refrigerated in an airtight glass jar for up to 2 weeks. Poach more salmon with it as many times as you want. With each use, the oil's fish flavor will become more pronounced. You can also use the oil in a Caesar vinaigrette for a nice anchovy-free dressing.

My method for cooking salmon ensures crisp skin and a moist medium-rare center, infused with the scent of lemon and dill. You can double the quantities below if you'd like. Just be sure to start with a very large pan or work in batches. You don't want to overcrowd the skillet, or the salmon skin won't brown. I like serving this over Sautéed Asparagus, Spring Onions, Artichokes, and Greens (page 102). It's also great over green salads or quinoa.

SERVES 2

PERFECTLY PAN-ROASTED SALMON

4 (6-ounce) thick skin-on wild salmon fillets

Coarse sea salt and freshly ground black pepper

Avocado oil

4 dill sprigs, torn

½ lemon

2 tablespoons grass-fed unsalted butter

1 Before you start cooking, pick out all the pin bones from the salmon with fish tweezers.

2 Preheat the oven to 375°F.

3 Season the skin side of the fish with salt and the flesh side with salt and pepper.

4 Heat a cast-iron skillet over medium-high heat. Coat the skillet with a thin layer of avocado oil. Add the salmon, skin-side down. Cook for 1 minute, pressing on the flesh side of the fish to prevent the whole thing from buckling. Lift the fillets and put them back down to help all the skin be in contact with the skillet so that it will brown evenly. Reduce the heat to medium and cook for 3 minutes.

RECIPE CONTINUES ▶

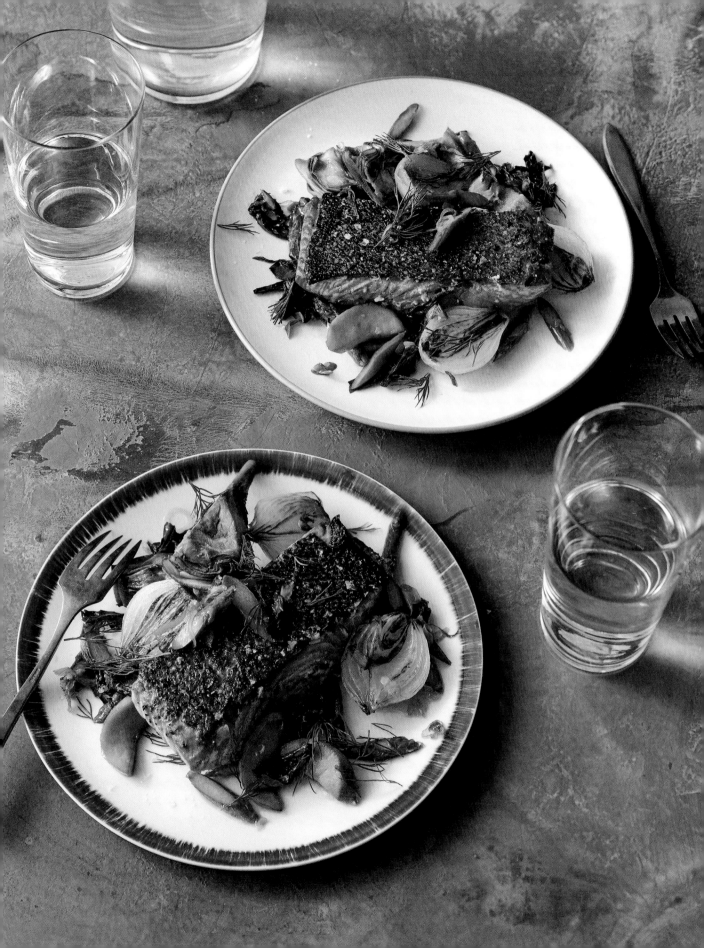

5 Remove from the heat and press the dill into the flesh, then zest the lemon on top. Top each fillet with ½ tablespoon of the butter. At this point, the flesh should be halfway to opaque. Transfer the skillet to the oven.

6 Roast until a metal cake tester or thin-bladed knife slipped into the thickest part of the fillet comes out warm, about 4 minutes. Put on serving plates skin-side up.

TECHNIQUE TIP: Salmon flesh should never come in contact with the cooking surface because the fat will oxidize and dry up. Let the skin take the heat and crisp in the process, too.

Ceviche, a South and Central American dish of fish cured in an acidic mixture, is a staple on fancy restaurant menus, but I prefer to not treat it with so much ceremony. It's actually a really easy dish to make—and enjoy—quickly. Here, sweet scallops get a nice punch from garlic that's mellowed by olive oil. Cucumber brings crunch and avocado lends creaminess. The only secret to this dish is to find the freshest scallops possible. If you live near a source of bay scallops and can buy them the day they're harvested, go for it. Otherwise, look for day-boat, dry-packed sea scallops.

SERVES 2

SCALLOP CEVICHE WITH LIME, CHILE, MINT, AND BASIL

I garlic clove

2 tablespoons extra-virgin olive oil

8 ounces very large sea scallops, tough muscles removed and discarded

4 cherry or grape tomatoes, preferably Sun Golds, cut into sixths

½ lime

I tablespoon very thinly sliced red finger chile

Jacobsen flake finishing sea salt

½ avocado, peeled and diced

¼ cucumber, peeled, seeded, and diced

3 tablespoons chopped fresh cilantro

I scallion, white part only, very thinly sliced

1   Grate just a tiny pinch of garlic, about $\frac{1}{16}$ teaspoon, into a medium bowl. Add the olive oil and stir well.

2   Thinly slice the scallops from top to bottom. Add to the garlic oil along with the tomatoes and squeeze in the lime juice. Reserve the lime rind. Toss well until everything is evenly coated.

3   Add the chile and a pinch of salt and stir well. Add the avocado, cucumber, cilantro, and scallion and fold gently. Zest the lime on top. Cover and refrigerate until cold, about 20 minutes.

4   Fold again and serve cold.

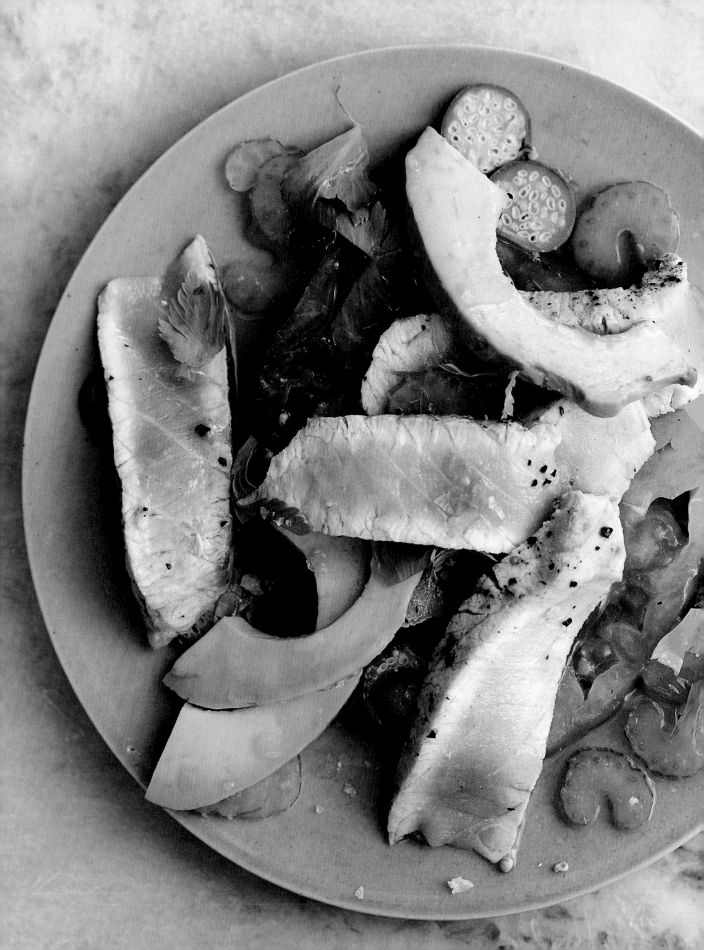

Swordfish is so much nicer when it's barely medium-rare. Usually, it's grilled over heat that's too high, leaving it dry. Ideally, you want just a quarter-inch rim of cooked fish around the rare center. To reinforce that moisture in the middle, I serve it over tomato slices that serve almost as plates. Together with the addition of celery, caper berries, and avocado, you get good fats, good protein, low carbs, and low sugar in a really tasty meal.

SERVES 4

SEARED SWORDFISH WITH HEIRLOOM TOMATOES, AVOCADO, CELERY, AND CAPER BERRIES

4 large heirloom tomatoes, thinly sliced

2 celery stalks, very thinly sliced crosswise, celery leaves reserved

8 caper berries, stemmed and very thinly sliced crosswise

Coarse sea salt and freshly ground black pepper

1 lemon

Extra-virgin olive oil

2 (10-ounce) swordfish steaks (1½ inches thick)

1 avocado, pitted, peeled, and thinly sliced

1   Divide the tomato slices among four serving plates and scatter the sliced celery and caper berries on top. Sprinkle with salt and pepper, then zest the lemon directly on top and drizzle with olive oil.

2   Heat a large cast-iron skillet over high heat. Coat the bottom of the skillet with olive oil. Season the fish with salt and pepper, then place it in the hot pan. Cook until golden brown, 2 to 3 minutes per side. The fish should be rare in the center. Transfer to a cutting board and let rest for a few minutes.

3   Cut the fish into ¼-inch-thick slices and scatter them over the vegetables, along with the avocado. Tear the reserved celery leaves and scatter them on top, then drizzle with olive oil. Serve immediately.

Meaty halibut takes well to grilling, especially when generously coated with olive oil. That prevents it from sticking to the grate and enriches the lean fish. In the summer, I like to serve it with Cherry Tomato, Anchovy, Basil, and Pistachio Sauce (page 300) for a delicious light, nutritious, and easy dinner.

SERVES 4

PERFECTLY GRILLED HALIBUT

4 (5-ounce) wild halibut fillets

Coarse sea salt and freshly ground black pepper

2 lemons

Extra-virgin olive oil

1 Heat a grill to medium-high.

2 Season the fish on all sides with salt and pepper. Zest the lemons directly over the fish, lightly covering the flesh with the zest. Very generously coat the fish with olive oil.

3 Grill the halibut until the flesh releases easily, then flip and grill the other side, about 2 minutes per side. Transfer to serving plates.

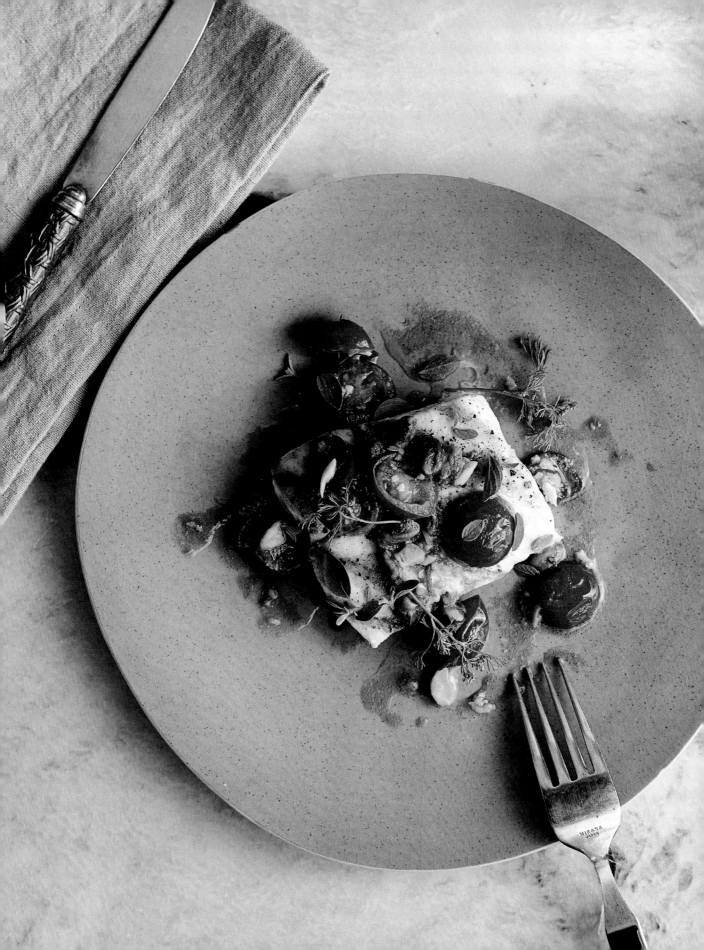

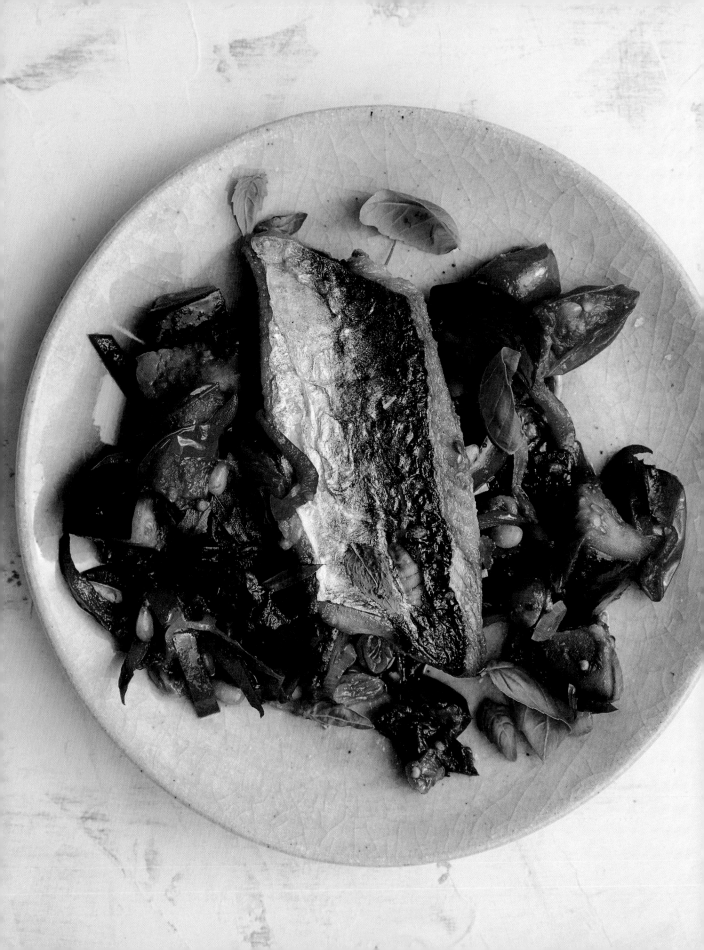

Mackerel is an oily, dark-fleshed fish, making it ideal for the sweet-and-sour richness of caponata. You can substitute bluefish or any other full-flavored fish, such as bonito, in this dish.

PAN-SEARED MACKEREL IN CAPONATA

Fresh and Dried Tomato Caponata (page 112)

4 (6-ounce) skin-on mackerel fillets

Coarse sea salt and freshly ground black pepper

Extra-virgin olive oil

Fresh basil leaves

1 If you've just made the caponata, keep it over low heat in the skillet. If you've made it ahead of time, put it in a large skillet and bring it to a simmer, stirring often, then keep it warm over low heat.

2 Generously season the fish fillets with salt and pepper.

3 Heat a large skillet over medium-high heat. Generously coat the bottom of the skillet with olive oil. When it's hot, add the fillets, skin-side down, working in batches if needed to avoid overcrowding the pan. Cook, without moving the fillets, until the skin is very browned and crisp and releases easily from the skillet, about 6 minutes.

4 Carefully transfer the fillets to the skillet with the caponata, arranging them in a single layer skin-side up. Nestle the fish in the warm caponata and let sit until a metal cake tester or thin-bladed knife inserted into the center of a fillet comes out warm, about 6 minutes.

5 Tear the basil leaves and scatter them on top, drizzle with oil, and serve immediately.

Talk about a one-pot powerhouse. You've got proteins, vegetables, and good fats all in one warming and delicious dish. Even though there isn't curry powder in the dish, it tastes like a curry, with its blend of coconut milk, lemongrass, ginger, and fish sauce. Keeping out the spice highlights the delicate sea-sweetness of the fish, scallops, and mussels.

SERVES 4

COCONUT SEAFOOD CURRY

2 tablespoons coconut oil

8 ounces monkfish, cut into 1-inch-thick medallions

8 very large sea scallops, tough muscles removed and discarded

Coarse sea salt and freshly ground black pepper

½ kabocha squash, seeded and cut into 1-inch wedges

2 carrots, cut into 1-inch pieces

1 trumpet royale mushroom, cut into 1-inch pieces

1 lemongrass stalk, lightly smashed with the back of a knife

1½ teaspoons rice vinegar

1 (13.5-ounce) can coconut milk

½ teaspoon fish sauce

1 shallot, sliced

1 baby bok choy, halved lengthwise

1 serrano chile, seeded, if desired, and thinly sliced

2 garlic cloves, sliced

1 (1-inch) piece fresh ginger, peeled and cut into thin slivers

12 ounces mussels, scrubbed and debearded

1 avocado, pitted, peeled, and diced

1 bunch scallions, trimmed and thinly sliced

Fresh cilantro and mint leaves, torn

Lime wedges

1 In a large Dutch oven or heavy saucepot, heat 1 tablespoon of the coconut oil over high heat. Season the monkfish and scallops with salt and pepper and place them in the hot pan, working in batches if needed to prevent overcrowding. Cook, turning once, until nicely seared, about 1 minute per side. Transfer to a plate.

2 Add the remaining 1 tablespoon oil, then the squash and carrots. Cook, stirring occasionally, until browned, about 5 minutes. Add the mushroom and lemongrass and cook, stirring often, until the vegetables are starting to soften, about 5 minutes.

RECIPE CONTINUES ▶

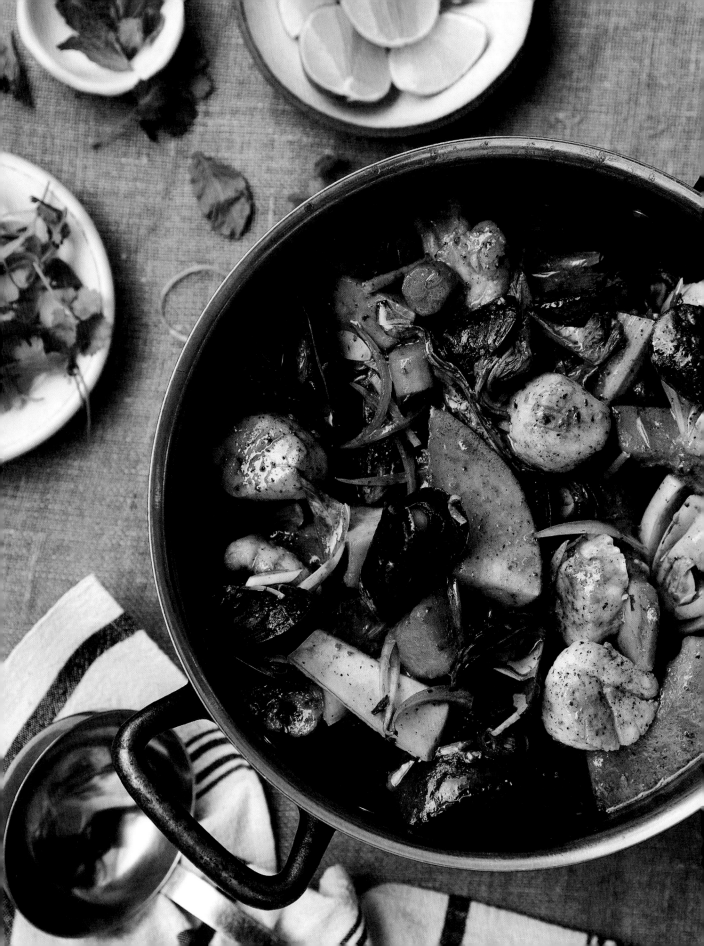

3 Add the vinegar and cook, stirring, until it has evaporated. Add the coconut milk and fish sauce. Season with salt and pepper, then reduce the heat to maintain a simmer and cook until the vegetables are tender, about 10 minutes.

4 Remove and discard the lemongrass. Add the shallot and seared monkfish and scallops and gently poach for a minute or two. Add the bok choy, chile, garlic, ginger, and mussels. Cover and steam until the mussels have opened, 3 to 5 minutes.

5 Uncover and season with salt and pepper. Divide among serving dishes and top with the avocado, scallions, cilantro, and mint. Serve immediately, with lime wedges for squeezing.

A bright ginger-herb sauce coating monkfish fillets stays vibrant when wrapped in gently steamed collard leaves. Steaming the bundles keeps the fish incredibly moist while trapping loads of flavor. Wrapping the fish is easy enough for a weeknight meal, but the finished dish looks impressive enough for a dinner party.

STEAMED PISTOU-RUBBED MONKFISH FILLETS WRAPPED IN COLLARDS

3 slices fresh ginger (unpeeled)

I tablespoon rice vinegar

2 large collard leaves

4 (5-ounce) monkfish fillets (4 inches long each), silver skin and red veins removed

Coarse sea salt and freshly ground black pepper

Ginger, Mint, Cilantro, and Basil Pistou with Coconut Oil (page 294)

Jacobsen flake finishing sea salt

1   Fill the bottom of a steamer with water to a depth of 1 inch. Add the ginger and vinegar and bring to a boil.

2   Cut off and discard the bottoms of the collard leaves, including the tough stems. Put the leaves in the steamer and steam until just bright green and tender, about 1 minute. Transfer to a cutting board and cool. Cut each leaf in half along the central rib, then cut out and discard the rib. You should now have four large pieces of steamed collards. Lay one piece flat on the cutting board.

3   Season a monkfish fillet with coarse sea salt and pepper, then brush a quarter of the pistou all over the fish to generously coat. Place the fillet on the collard, matching the long side of the fish to the long side

RECIPE CONTINUES ▶

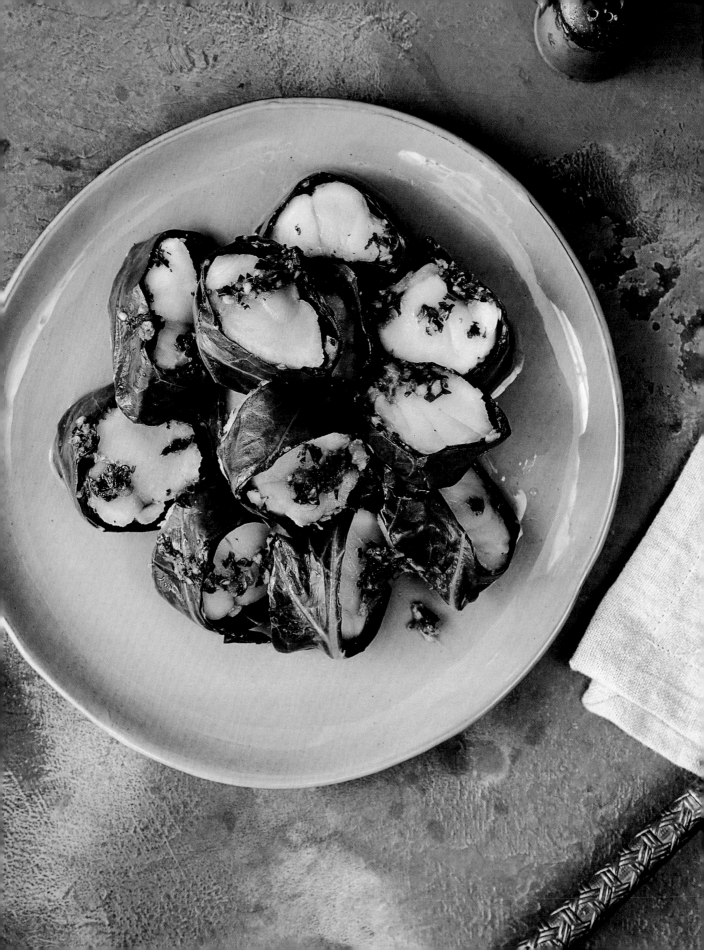

of the leaf, leaving a 3-inch rim from the long edge. Fold that long edge over the fish, then fold in the sides and roll up tightly. Repeat with the remaining monkfish, pistou, and collards.

4   Check the steamer and replenish the water if needed. Bring to a rolling boil. Place the wrapped fish in the steamer and steam until a metal cake tester or thin-bladed knife inserted into the center of the fish comes out almost hot, about 6 minutes. Transfer to a clean cutting board.

5   Cut the fish into 1-inch slices at an angle. Sprinkle with finishing salt and serve immediately.

TECHNIQUE TIP: Whenever I steam something, I always put some aromatics in the liquid to give it flavor.

If you don't have a steamer, you can improvise one: Set a small wire rack or ramekins or a dish placed upside-down in a large, wide saucepan with a lid. Fill the pan with ½ inch of water and bring to a simmer. Put the wrapped fish on a heatproof plate and balance it on the rack, ramekins, or plate. Cover and steam until cooked through.

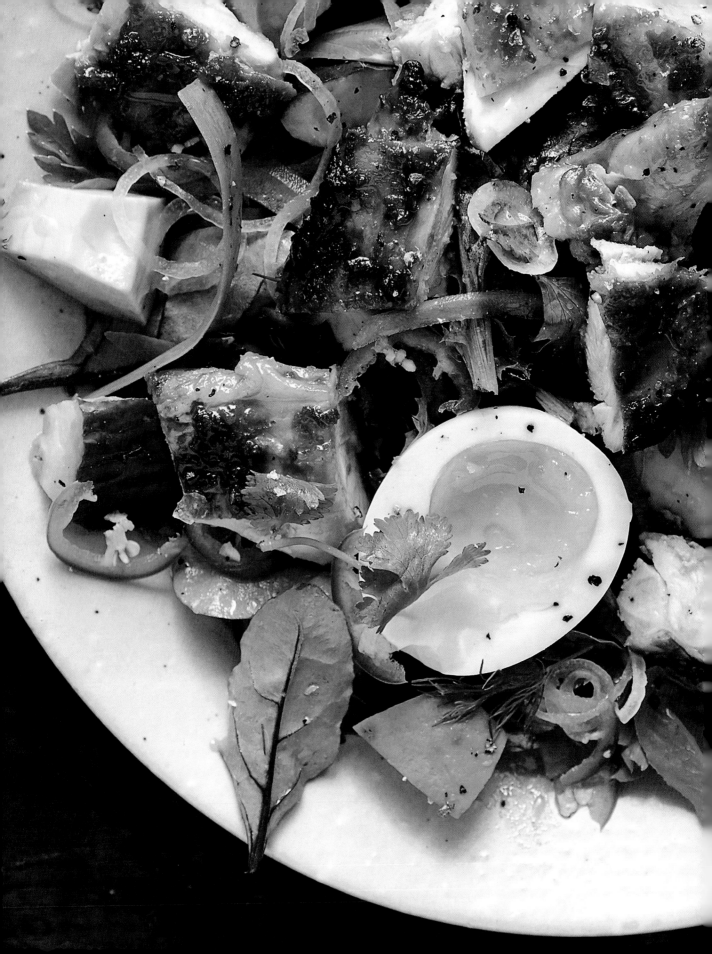

CHICKEN

In the real world, chicken is a universally liked protein. In chef world, it can be perceived as a little boring. Even though I'm a chef, I can't think of anything more comforting than a good braised chicken. My grandmother Mutti would do a one-pot chicken braise with white wine, leeks, and carrots. It's still one of my favorite dishes, and the inspiration behind my braises (pages 215 to 221). Nostalgia aside, I think a perfectly prepared chicken tastes as good as anything else. When the meat is succulent, it's indulgent and works with a huge variety of vegetables and seasonings.

From an environmental standpoint, ethically raising chickens naturally has a much lower carbon footprint than what's required with other animals. Chickens have a quick life cycle because they mature quickly, so they require less energy to raise on a calorie-by-calorie basis. If they're raised properly and sustainably, they'll fertilize the soil, too. As a bonus, chickens produce incredibly delicious eggs and are a healthy source of both protein and natural fat.

The difference between factory-farmed and free-range birds is tremendous in both the quality of the product and the life of the animal. As with all animal pro-teins, I always try to consume it consciously and with knowledge of where it's com-ing from. For me, that means buying chickens from small farms I trust that allow their chickens to openly roam pasture.

From a nutritional standpoint, chicken is a relatively lean healthy protein. It's still got some good fat on it, which is extremely important for overall nutrition, so I like to keep the skin on whenever I'm preparing it. That it's delicious doesn't hurt, either.

When I want to really impress with my roast chicken, I brine it first. It keeps the meat incredibly juicy while infusing it with spices, herbs, and citrus. Since it's sort of a lengthy and involved process, I do two at a time.

BRINED ROAST CHICKENS

I cup kosher salt

⅔ cup raw honey

I tablespoon whole black peppercorns

I tablespoon coriander seeds

I teaspoon fennel seeds

5 thyme sprigs

I rosemary sprig

I bay leaf

Zest of I orange, removed with a vegetable peeler

Zest of I lemon, removed with a vegetable peeler

2 (2- to 3-pound) whole free-range sustainably raised chickens

Coarse sea salt and freshly ground black pepper

Extra-virgin olive oil

1   In a large saucepot, combine the kosher salt, honey, peppercorns, coriander, fennel, thyme, rosemary, bay leaf, orange zest, lemon zest, and 8 cups water. Heat over high heat, stirring until the salt has dissolved completely. Remove from the heat and add 8 cups cold water. Let cool completely, stirring occasionally.

2   Put the chickens in a large container that holds them snugly and strain the brine over them. Discard the solids in the strainer. Cover and refrigerate for 3 hours. (If you don't have room in your fridge for the chickens in the brine, you can put the birds in a clean garbage bag and pour in the brine. Tie the bag tightly and put it in an insulated cooler with a lot of ice or ice packs.)

3   Fit a wire rack into a rimmed baking sheet or line the baking sheet with paper towels. Remove the chickens from the brine and place them on the rack. Refrigerate, uncovered, overnight to let the birds air-dry.

4   Preheat the oven to 400°F.

5   Lightly season the chickens with sea salt and pepper and rub with olive oil. Place the chickens, breast-side up, on a rimmed baking sheet, spacing them apart.

6   Roast until an instant-read thermometer inserted into the inside of the thigh joint (but not hitting bone) registers 155°F, 45 minutes to 1 hour.

7   Transfer to a cutting board to rest and cool slightly, at least 15 minutes. Chow down on one bird; shred the meat of the other with a fork and refrigerate for other uses.

I roast two chickens at a time so I can use them for lots of meals. I'll have some for dinner the night I roast them, then pull the remaining meat off to use for meals for the rest of the week. A little bit of prep goes a long way to making weekday cooking easy. Even the night I'm cooking the chickens, I'll prep a salad and vegetables while the birds are in the oven. The next day, I'll throw some leftovers over quinoa with Caesar dressing or into a green salad.

BASIC ROAST CHICKENS

| 2 (2- to 3-pound) whole free-range sustainably raised chickens | Coarse sea salt and freshly ground black pepper | Chopped mixed fresh herbs, such as thyme, rosemary, and sage |

1 Preheat the oven to 425°F.

2 Generously season the chickens inside and out with salt and pepper. Stuff the cavities of the birds with herbs, then truss the chickens, tying their legs and wings against their bodies with kitchen twine. Place the chickens on a rimmed baking sheet, breast-side up, spacing them apart.

3 Roast until an instant-read thermometer inserted into the inside of the thigh joint (but not hitting bone) registers 155°F, 45 minutes to 1 hour.

4 Transfer to a cutting board to rest and cool slightly, at least 15 minutes. Chow down on one bird; shred the meat of the other with a fork and refrigerate for other uses.

Chicken skewers are often grilled, but searing them results in even more browning. And that's where the flavor is. Just be sure to use skewers that are shorter than the diameter of your pan. Even though the turmeric-and-coriander-marinated chicken tastes great on its own, it's even better when served with Gingered Cucumber Kefir Raita (page 292) for dipping.

SERVES
4 TO 6

SEARED KEFIR-MARINATED CHICKEN AND TOMATO SKEWERS

2 cups plain full-fat kefir

1 tablespoon finely grated fresh turmeric

1 tablespoon ground coriander

Zest of 1 lemon

2 pounds chicken thighs

4 cups cherry tomatoes

Coarse sea salt and freshly ground black pepper

Avocado oil

In a large bowl, combine the kefir, turmeric, coriander, and lemon zest. Debone the chicken by running a sharp knife along the bones to create a slit, exposing the bones. Open the slits and slide the knife under the bones to scrape the meat away and release the bones. Save the bones for another use. Cut the meat into 1- by 2-inch pieces. Place in the marinade and turn to coat. Cover and refrigerate for at least 4 hours and up to overnight.

Remove the chicken from the marinade; discard the marinade. Thread a chicken piece onto a skewer by folding the piece in half so the skin side is facing out on all sides. Thread a tomato onto the skewer. Repeat with the remaining chicken and tomatoes, alternating pieces on skewers. Generously season with salt and pepper.

In a large cast-iron skillet, heat enough avocado oil to coat the bottom of the skillet over medium-high heat, swirling to coat. Cook the skewers, turning to evenly brown them, for about 10 minutes total.

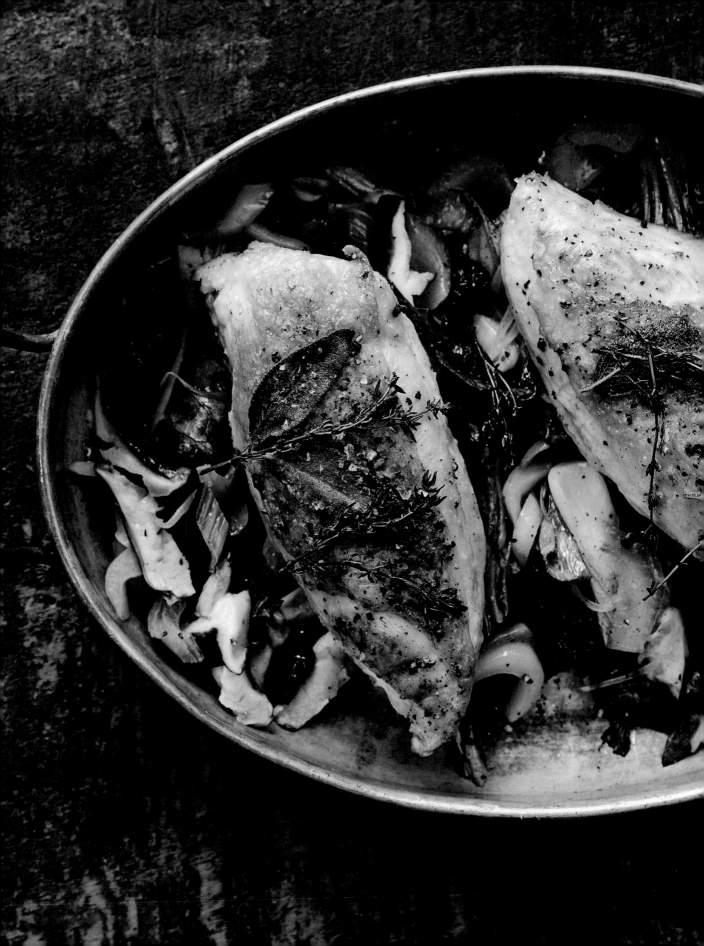

Some chefs scorn chicken breasts. I'm not one of them. I think they can be succulent if cooked gently. If they get hammered, they're not nice, to put it mildly. But follow the technique below and you'll end up with chicken worth savoring. I especially like it with Stir-Fried Bok Choy and Shiitakes (page 105).

PERFECT PAN-ROASTED CHICKEN BREAST

I whole bone-in, skin-on chicken breast (about 1¼ pounds)

Kosher salt and freshly ground black pepper

I lemon

Extra-virgin olive oil

6 thyme sprigs

3 sage sprigs

I tablespoon grass-fed unsalted butter, cut into pieces

Preheat the oven to 400°F.

Generously season the chicken breast on all sides with salt and pepper. Zest half the lemon directly onto the chicken skin, then drizzle with olive oil.

Heat a medium cast-iron skillet over medium-high heat. Coat the bottom of the pan with oil. When the oil is hot but not smoking, add the chicken, skin-side down. Cook, without moving it, until the skin is nicely browned, about 2 minutes.

Turn the chicken with tongs and hold the side of it against the pan for 1 minute, then repeat on the other side. Transfer the chicken to a rimmed baking sheet, skin-side up. Press the thyme and sage onto the chicken skin, then scatter the butter over the herbs. Zest a quarter of the lemon on top.

Roast until an instant-read thermometer inserted into the thickest part registers 150°F, about 20 minutes. Transfer to a cutting board and let rest for 5 to 10 minutes.

Panzanella is a traditional Italian salad made with fat cubes of bread. Swapping in chicken chunks makes the dish even more satisfying and flavorful. The addition of watermelon keeps it feeling light, and a surprising saffron dressing delivers aromatic notes. I make a huge batch of this because it's perfect for parties. You can halve the recipe if you're cooking for a smaller crowd.

SERVES 8 TO 10

ROASTED CHICKEN AND HEIRLOOM TOMATO "PANZANELLA" WITH PECANS AND HERBS

2 Brined Roast Chickens (page 200), cut into 1-inch chunks

4 very large heirloom tomatoes, cored and cut into 1-inch chunks

1 cup watermelon chunks (about 1 inch each)

1 watermelon radish, cut into paper-thin slices with a mandoline

½ cup pecans, toasted

¼ cup thinly sliced garlic scapes

1 shallot, cut into paper-thin rings with a mandoline, rings separated

Jacobsen flake finishing sea salt

Saffron Vinaigrette (recipe follows)

Fresh mint, thyme, basil, tarragon, and parsley leaves

1   In a large bowl, combine the chicken, tomatoes, watermelon, watermelon radish, pecans, garlic scapes, and shallot. Season with salt and toss well. Drizzle with the vinaigrette and toss until everything is evenly coated.

2   Divide among serving dishes and top with the herbs. Serve immediately.

RECIPE CONTINUES ▶

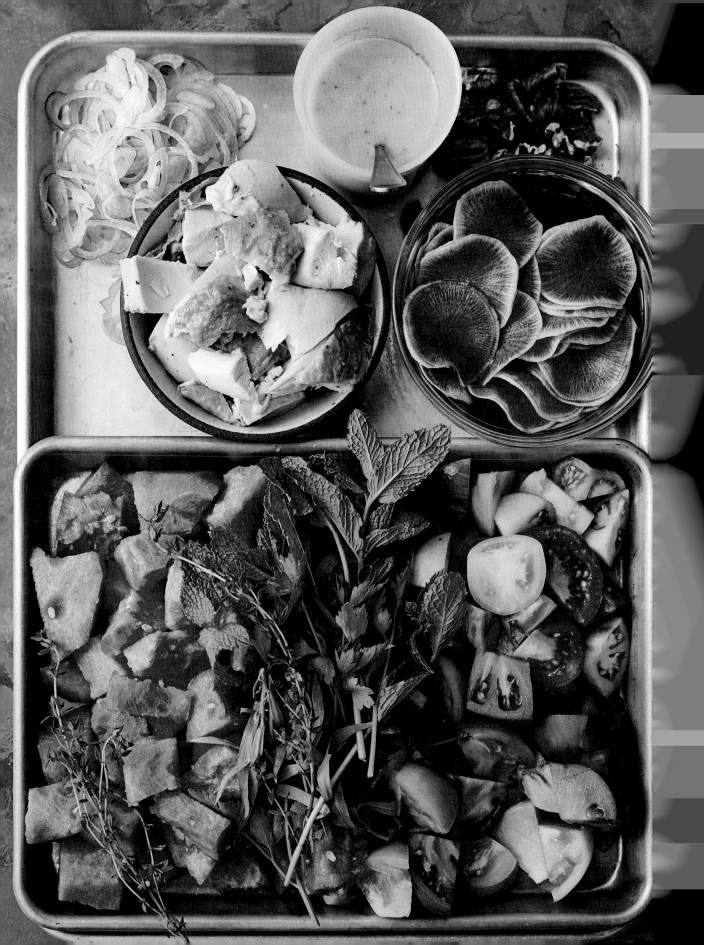

SAFFRON VINAIGRETTE MAKES ABOUT ½ CUP

2½ tablespoons raw apple cider vinegar

2 saffron threads

½ teaspoon raw honey

¼ garlic clove, grated on a Microplane

¼ teaspoon whole-grain Dijon mustard

⅓ cup extra-virgin olive oil

Coarse sea salt and freshly ground black pepper

In a small bowl, whisk together the vinegar, saffron, honey, garlic, and mustard until smooth. While whisking, add the olive oil in a slow, steady stream. Whisk until emulsified. Season with salt and pepper.

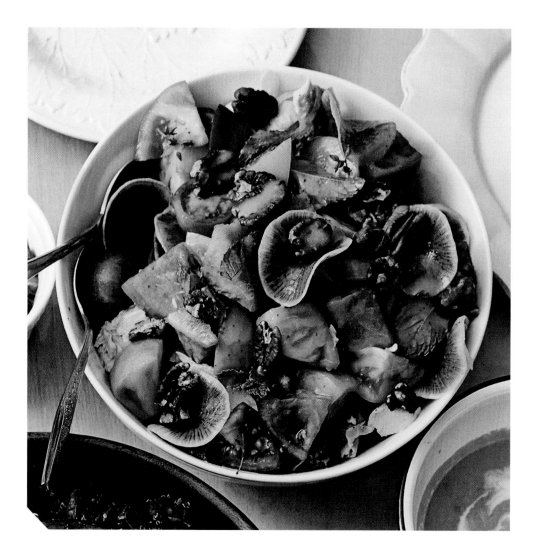

This is a healthy lunch salad with a perfect balance of protein, carbs, fat, and vegetables. It takes a little prep ahead of time, so I like to do most of the heavy lifting the night before. This means cooking the quinoa, chicken, and eggs in the evening as well as preparing the vinaigrette. The next day, you can simply assemble the salad before bringing it to work for lunch or quickly throw it together for dinner at night.

SERVES
1 OR 2

KALE AND CHICKEN CAESAR SALAD WITH QUINOA AND PECANS

1 cup Aromatic Tricolor Quinoa (page 307)

1 cup coarsely shredded cooked Basic Roast Chickens (page 202)

2 cups mixed kale, finely chopped

1 avocado, pitted, peeled, halved, and cut into slices

1 apple, cored and thinly sliced

¼ cup pecans, toasted

Coarse sea salt and freshly ground black pepper

¼ cup Caesar Vinaigrette (recipe follows)

1 Just-Right Boiled Egg (page 306), peeled and halved lengthwise

1   In a large bowl, combine the quinoa, chicken, kale, avocado, apple, and pecans in a large bowl. Season with salt and pepper and toss well. Add the vinaigrette and toss until everything is well coated.

2   To pack for lunch, transfer the salad to an airtight container and top with the egg. Seal and chill until it's time to eat. Otherwise, top with the egg and enjoy right away .

RECIPE CONTINUES ▶

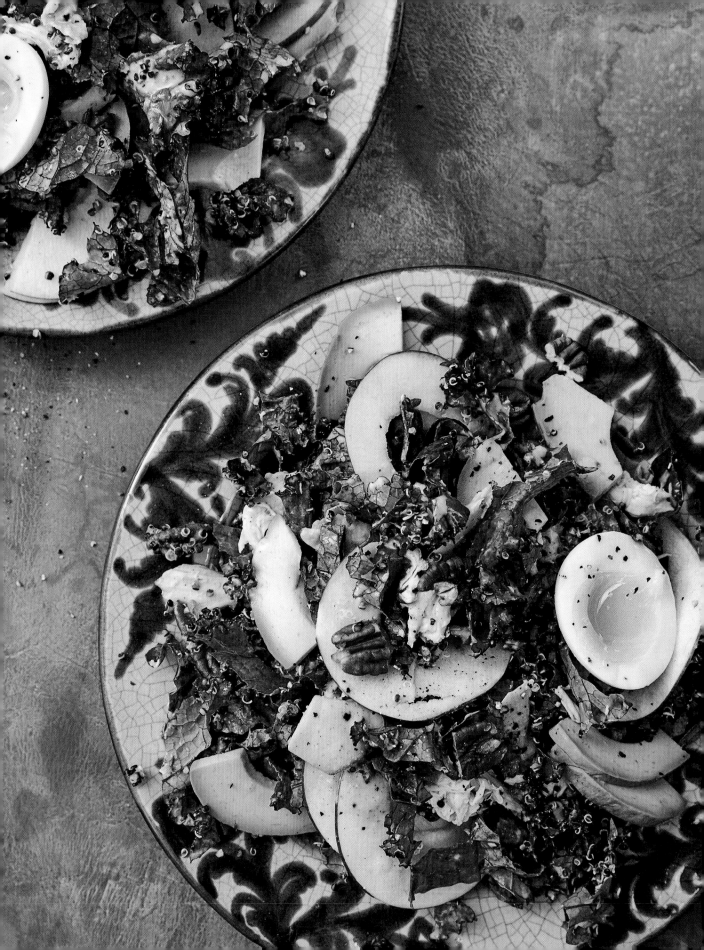

CAESAR VINAIGRETTE MAKES ABOUT ¾ CUP

3 tablespoons white wine vinegar

½ garlic clove

1 anchovy fillet

½ teaspoon Dijon mustard

½ teaspoon raw honey

Zest and juice of ½ lemon

Leaves from 1 tarragon sprig

Coarse sea salt and freshly ground black pepper

1 tablespoon grated Parmesan cheese (optional)

½ cup extra-virgin olive oil

1 In a blender, combine the vinegar, garlic, anchovy, mustard, honey, lemon zest, lemon juice, tarragon, a pinch each of salt and pepper, and the Parmesan, if using. Puree until very smooth.

2 With the machine running on a slow setting, add the olive oil in a thin, steady stream and blend until emulsified. Use immediately or transfer to a jar and refrigerate for up to 2 weeks. Bring to room temperature before using.

Southeast Asian flavors run through this nice contrast of hot chicken over cold salad. They're bound together by the marinade, which is boiled after seasoning the chicken so it can be turned into the salad dressing. I like chicken legs because of the different textures of the thigh and drumstick, but I also like deboning them so they cook more evenly. You can save the bones for stock (see page 139).

SERVES 4

TAMARI-GLAZED CHICKEN SALAD WITH AVOCADO, PEPITAS, AND HARD-BOILED EGGS

GLAZED CHICKEN

⅓ cup reduced-sodium gluten-free tamari

¼ cup rice vinegar

2 tablespoons pure maple syrup

I tablespoon fish sauce

I tablespoon cayenne hot sauce

I garlic clove, grated on a Microplane

I (I-inch) piece fresh ginger, grated on a Microplane

I (½-inch) piece fresh turmeric, grated on a Microplane

Zest of ¼ lemon

4 chicken legs

SALAD

5 ounces spring mix

½ shallot, very thinly sliced

½ English cucumber, cut into ¾-inch chunks

I avocado, pitted, peeled, and cut into I-inch chunks

2 carrots, scrubbed and shaved into ribbons with a vegetable peeler

½ bunch cilantro, torn into bite-size pieces

I serrano or jalapeño chile, very thinly sliced

3 tablespoons pepitas (hulled pumpkin seeds)

Jacobsen flake finishing sea salt

Juice of 2 limes

2 Just-Right Boiled Eggs (page 306), peeled and halved lengthwise (optional)

To make the glazed chicken, in a shallow dish that will hold the chicken snugly, combine the tamari, vinegar, maple syrup, fish sauce, hot sauce, garlic, ginger, turmeric, and lemon zest. Debone the chicken legs by running a sharp knife along the bones to create a slit, exposing

RECIPE CONTINUES ▶

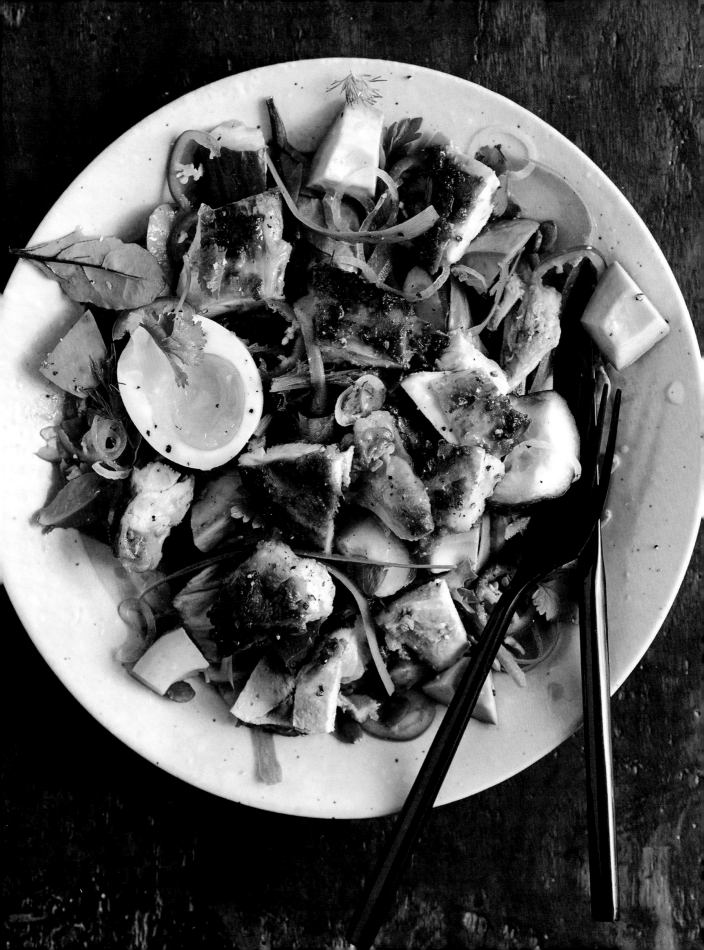

the bones. Open the slits and slide the knife under the bones to scrape the meat away and release the bones. Save the bones for another use. Add the chicken to the marinade and turn to coat. Cover and refrigerate for at least 30 minutes or up to 4 hours.

2   Preheat the oven to 375°F.

3   Place the chicken skin-side down in a single layer in a 9 by 13-inch glass or ceramic baking dish. Transfer the marinade to a small saucepan. Bake the chicken for 18 minutes; boil the marinade for 5 minutes. Turn the chicken over and brush with just enough of the boiled marinade to coat the skin. Turn the oven to broil and broil the chicken for 5 minutes.

4   While the chicken cooks, make the salad. In a large bowl, combine the spring mix, shallot, cucumber, avocado, carrots, cilantro, chile, and pepitas. Sprinkle with salt and toss to mix.

5   Add the lime juice to the marinade and whisk well. Drizzle over the salad and toss until well coated. Divide the salad among serving dishes and top each with an egg half, if desired. Sprinkle the eggs with salt.

6   Cut the chicken into 1-inch chunks and scatter the hot pieces over the salad. Drizzle any juices from the baking dish over the chicken. Serve immediately.

One-pot meals are the best. I'm a big fan of having everything I crave in a single pot, and find a deep comfort in that style of cooking and eating. If you happen to have any of this stew left over, it makes for a great breakfast or lunch the following day.

SERVES 4 TO 6

BRAISED CHICKEN AND QUINOA STEW WITH MUSHROOMS AND WINTER GREENS

¼ cup dried shiitake mushrooms

2 cups boiling water

¼ cup extra-virgin olive oil

4 organic or free-range chicken legs

1 tablespoon Chinese five-spice powder

Coarse sea salt and freshly ground black pepper

4 shallots, halved lengthwise

1 cup 1-inch pieces king oyster mushrooms

2 garlic cloves, thinly sliced

½ cup Chinese rice wine

1 cup tricolor quinoa, rinsed under cold running water and drained

1 tablespoon star anise pods

4 cups Chicken Stock (page 139) or store-bought unsalted chicken broth

2 cups coarsely chopped mustard greens or other winter greens

Put the dried shiitakes in a medium bowl and pour the boiling water over. Let stand for 25 minutes. Strain through a fine-mesh sieve into a bowl, reserving the soaking liquid and mushrooms separately.

In a large heavy-bottomed pot, heat the olive oil over medium-high heat. Season the chicken legs with the five-spice, salt, and pepper. Place them in the hot pan in a single layer, working in batches if needed to avoid overcrowding, and cook, turning once, until nicely browned, 5 to 6 minutes per side. Transfer to a plate.

RECIPE CONTINUES ▶

3   Add the shallots and king oyster mushrooms to the pan and cook, stirring often, for 2 minutes. Stir in the rehydrated shiitakes and the garlic, then add the wine. Cook, stirring and scraping the bottom of the pan, until the wine has cooked off, about 2 minutes.

4   Add the quinoa and return the chicken legs to the pan, along with any juices that have accumulated on the plate. Add the mushroom soaking liquid, star anise, and stock. Season with salt and pepper and bring to a boil. Cover, reduce the heat to low, and simmer until the chicken is tender and the quinoa is cooked through, about 25 minutes.

5   Add the mustard greens and cook, stirring occasionally, until tender, 5 to 7 minutes. Season with salt and pepper and serve.

MUSTARD GREENS

Mustard greens are anything but boring. They're spicy, with tender leaves and crisp stems. Bunches can be really dirty, so I like to wash them in a salad spinner, immersing them in cold water and lifting them out to get rid of all the grit before spinning them dry. Once they're ready, I don't like to cook them super hard and fast. Getting just enough heat on them to wilt them keeps their zing.

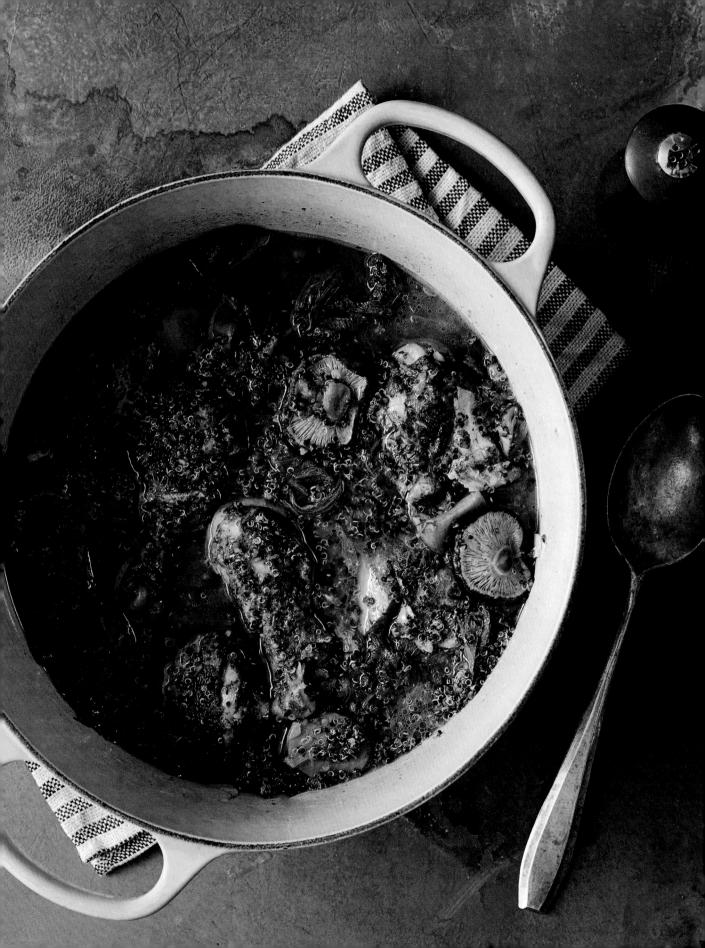

Braises end up being relegated to winter, but they're delicious in spring and summer, too. You get the benefit of tender, slowly cooked chicken along with fresh artichokes, carrots, squash, and green beans, which make the whole meal feel light.

SERVES
6 TO 8

MARKET VEGETABLE AND CHICKEN BRAISE

Extra-virgin olive oil

1 (3-pound) whole chicken, cut into 8 pieces

Coarse sea salt and freshly ground black pepper

2 artichokes, prepped (see page 38) and halved

4 spring garlic, white and pale green parts only, cut into 4-inch pieces, or 4 garlic cloves, peeled and kept whole

2 shallots, peeled and kept whole

2 carrots, cut into 2½-inch batons

2 tablespoons raw apple cider vinegar

1 cup dry white wine

6 thyme sprigs

1 bay leaf

4 cups Chicken Stock (page 139) or store-bought unsalted chicken broth, plus more if needed

2 summer squash, cut into 1-inch chunks

6 ounces green beans, trimmed and halved

Fresh flat-leaf parsley, chopped

1   In a large Dutch oven, heat enough olive oil to coat the bottom of the pan over medium-high heat. Generously season the chicken with salt and pepper. Place the chicken in the hot pan, skin-side down, working in batches if needed to avoid overcrowding the pan. Cook, turning the pieces to evenly brown them, until deeply seared, 8 to 10 minutes. Transfer to a plate.

2   Drain the artichokes and add them to the pan along with the spring garlic, shallots, and carrots. Season with salt and pepper. If the pan seems dry, add more oil. Cook, stirring often, until golden brown, about 6 minutes.

3   Return the chicken and any accumulated juices to the pan, then add the vinegar. Cook, stirring, until the vinegar has completely evaporated, then add the wine. Cook, stirring and scraping the pan, until the wine has reduced by half, then add the thyme, bay leaf, and stock. The stock should just cover the meat and vegetables. If it doesn't, add more.

4   Bring to a boil, then reduce the heat to low, cover partially, and simmer for 10 minutes. Add the squash and green beans, nestling them into the mixture, and cover the pan partially. Simmer until the meat is cooked through and all the vegetables are tender, 20 to 25 minutes. Remove and discard the bay leaf.

5   Season with salt and pepper. Sprinkle parsley on top, drizzle with olive oil, and serve hot.

This dish is loaded with antioxidants, has a balance of nutritious plant and animal proteins, and is packed with micronutrients. The micronutrients are made bioavailable with abundant healthy fats. Because this dish is naturally low in simple carbohydrates and sugar, it means no insulin spike, which means less stress on the hormonal system and no white fat production.

SERVES 4

BRAISED CHICKEN WITH SHIITAKE MUSHROOMS, BITTER GREENS, GINGER, AND COCONUT

¼ cup dried shiitake mushrooms

4 tablespoons coconut oil

4 chicken legs

1 tablespoon Chinese five-spice powder

Coarse sea salt and freshly ground black pepper

4 shallots, halved lengthwise

1 cup king oyster mushrooms, cut into 1-inch pieces

2 garlic cloves, thinly sliced

½ cup Chinese rice wine

1 cup tricolor quinoa, rinsed under cold running water and drained

1 tablespoon star anise pods

4 cups Chicken Stock (page 139) or store-bought unsalted chicken broth

2 cups mustard greens, dandelion greens, or kale leaves, coarsely chopped

2 tablespoons slivered peeled fresh ginger

1 teaspoon grated fresh turmeric

2 tablespoons unsweetened dried coconut flakes

1   Bring 2 cups water to a boil. Put the dried shiitakes in a small bowl. Pour the boiling water over the mushrooms and let stand for 25 minutes. Drain through a sieve into a bowl, reserving the mushrooms and their soaking liquid separately.

2   In a Dutch oven or large, heavy saucepot, heat the coconut oil over medium-high heat. Season the chicken with the five-spice and salt and pepper. Place the chicken in the hot pan, working in batches if needed to avoid overcrowding, and cook, turning once, until nicely browned, about 8 minutes. Transfer to a plate.

Add the shallots and king oyster mushrooms to the pan and cook, stirring often, for 2 minutes, then add the drained shiitake mushrooms and the garlic. Stir well, then add the wine. Cook, stirring, until the wine has cooked off, about 2 minutes.

Add the quinoa and the chicken, along with any juices that have accumulated on the plate, then add the mushroom soaking liquid, star anise, and stock. Season with salt and pepper. Bring to a boil, then reduce the heat to maintain a simmer, cover, and cook until the chicken is tender and the quinoa is cooked through, about 25 minutes. Stir in the greens, ginger, and turmeric. Simmer for 5 minutes. Season with salt and pepper.

Divide among serving dishes and top with the coconut flakes. Serve immediately.

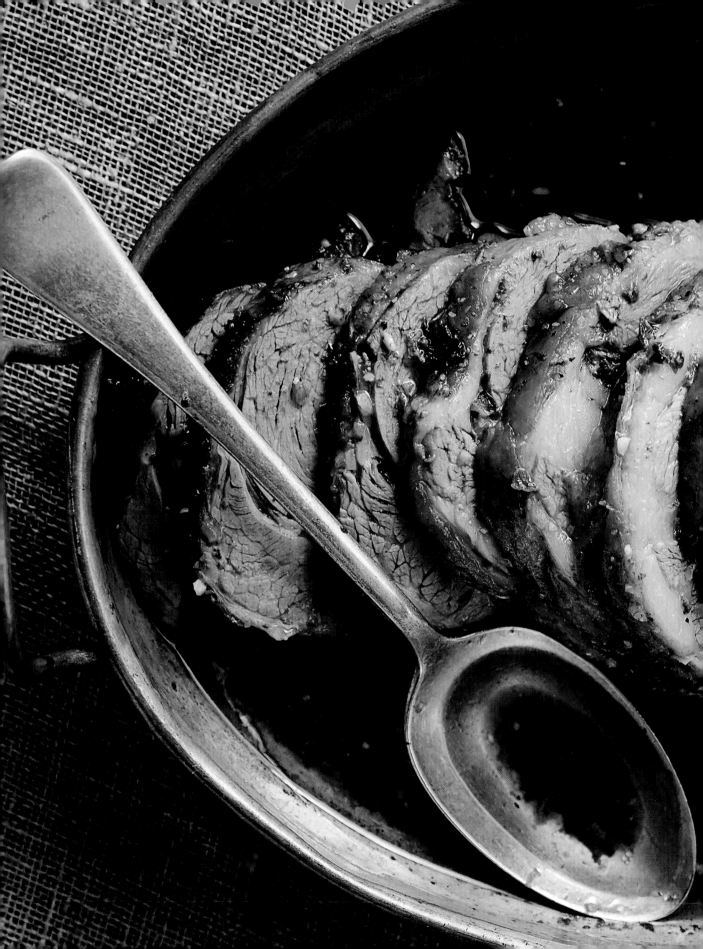

MEAT

There's something really homey and satisfying about carving into a roast or a grilled steak. There's a balance of both nostalgia and a kind of primal relationship with protein. We've been eating meat since we became bipeds. It's one of the things that differentiates us from primates. There's a reason why anytime you light a grill, crowds gather. Humans are drawn to fire—and not only because it's warming. There's something in our DNA that tells us that's where we gather. And fire and meat go hand in hand.

Despite that very real primal relationship to eating meat, my consumption has gone down, down, down over the years. I now treat it more as a seasoning than a main ingredient. For example, I'll break up a seared patty over a salad for lunch and then not have any more meat the rest of the day. In doing so, I'm striving for a more balanced relationship between protein and vegetables. We should reorient ourselves away from the traditional makeup of the plate to make vegetables the bulk of the meal and meat the accent.

This isn't to say I don't love cooking big cuts of meat. I do. In fact, cuts like lamb shoulder are better when prepared in large portions and then carved. It's just that I now share those big cuts with a crowd rather than giving one individual a gigantic hunk. For example, a single thick, bone-in pork chop can serve four people when there are a lot of vegetables to go around, too.

I found that when I started cutting back on my meat portion sizes and increasing my intake of fibrous and nutrient-dense vegetables, I didn't feel like anything was missing. On the contrary—I felt a lot better.

From a flavor standpoint, eating less meat also has its benefits. It's really easy to get palate fatigue with any ingredient, and we tend to overeat specific ingredients, such as meat. And then we feel overly full and bloated and have consumed far more than what we need in terms of calories. Consuming a smaller portion is the ideal for true pleasure when eating. As a chef, I want you to finish each dish wishing there was one more bite so you look forward to the next dish. If you have just enough, you'll more fully appreciate what you just had *and* what's to come.

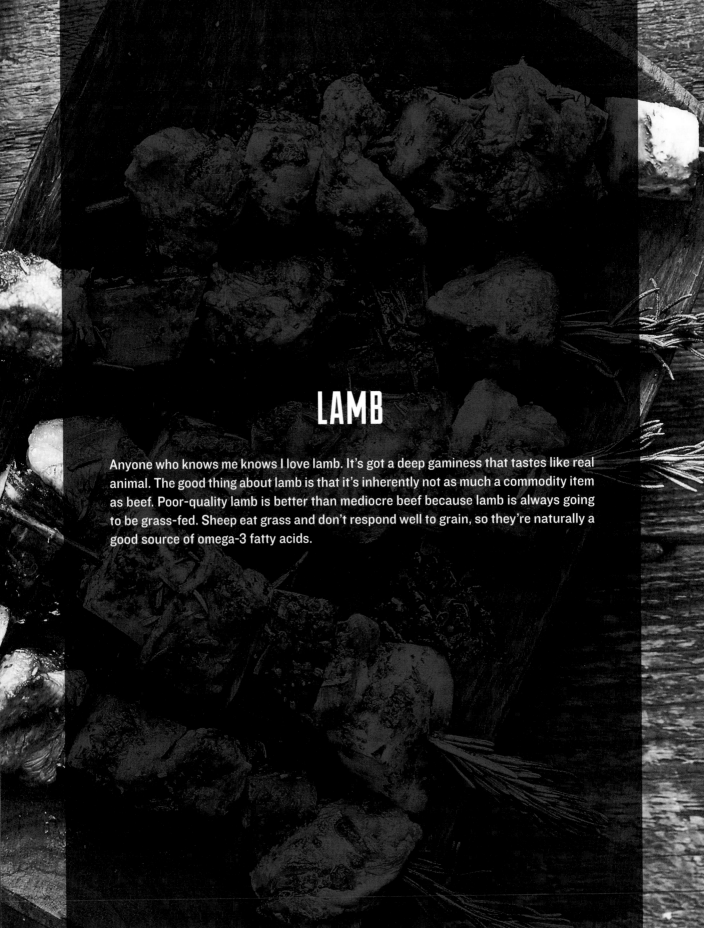

LAMB

Anyone who knows me knows I love lamb. It's got a deep gaminess that tastes like real animal. The good thing about lamb is that it's inherently not as much a commodity item as beef. Poor-quality lamb is better than mediocre beef because lamb is always going to be grass-fed. Sheep eat grass and don't respond well to grain, so they're naturally a good source of omega-3 fatty acids.

At my restaurants, I get whole lambs and break them down myself. It gives me control over the cuts. For example, I like leaving the thick layer of fat known as the deckle on the rib chops. Try to find untrimmed chops—that fat is so tasty. Here tart rhubarb cuts through the richness, as do bitter greens and woody mushrooms. Pomegranate molasses, which shouldn't have any added sugar, binds everything together with a Middle Eastern vibe. If you can't get untrimmed chops, use eight trimmed chops instead. Either way, you can finish the dish with Mint Yogurt Sauce (page 290).

SERVES 4

LAMB CHOPS WITH SHIITAKES AND RHUBARB

8 cipollini onions

¼ cup pomegranate molasses

¼ cup extra-virgin olive oil, plus more for cooking

I garlic clove, grated on a Microplane

7 thyme sprigs

Freshly ground black pepper

4 (6-ounce) untrimmed lamb rib chops

3½ tablespoons unsalted grass-fed butter

26 small shiitake mushroom caps

Coarse sea salt

I rhubarb stalk, tough fibers peeled off, cut into ¾-inch-thick slices

8 mustard or collard green leaves, ribs removed, cut into 2-inch-wide slices

Place the onions in a small bowl and cover with very hot (almost boiling) water. Let stand for 10 minutes.

RECIPE CONTINUES ▶

POMEGRANATE MOLASSES

Syrupy, with a tangy sweetness, true pomegranate molasses is made by simply boiling down pomegranate juice. Be sure there's no added sugar in the product you buy; the only ingredient should be pomegranates or pomegranate juice. I like the Al Wadi brand.

2   Meanwhile, in a shallow dish that will hold the lamb snugly, combine the molasses, olive oil, and garlic. Strip the thyme leaves off 5 sprigs, crushing them with your hands to release their oils, and add to the molasses mixture, along with a generous grinding of pepper. Add the lamb chops and turn to coat. Let stand until ready to cook.

3   Drain the onions and trim the tops and bottoms, then quarter them. Peel off and discard the outer skins. In a large cast-iron skillet, melt 2 tablespoons of the butter over medium heat. Add the onions and swirl them around in the melted butter, then add the shiitakes in a single layer, gill-side down, and top with the remaining 2 thyme sprigs. Let stand for 1 minute, then toss well and turn the mushrooms gill-side up. Season with salt. Cook, stirring occasionally, until the mushrooms are tender, about 4 minutes.

4   Add the remaining 1½ tablespoons butter and the rhubarb and stir well. Pour in the lamb marinade, leaving the lamb behind, and season the rhubarb mixture with salt and pepper. Cook, stirring occasionally, until the rhubarb is just tender, about 3 minutes. Add the greens and cook, stirring, until just wilted, about 1 minute. Season with salt, then transfer to a serving platter.

5   While the rhubarb and greens cook, heat another large cast-iron skillet over medium-high heat. Season the lamb generously with salt and pepper. Place the lamb in the skillet fat-side down, arranging the chops right next to one another so they can stand on their curved tops. Cook until charred and the fat has rendered, 1 to 2 minutes. Turn the chops onto their flat sides and cook until nicely charred on both sides, 2 to 3 minutes per side. Place on top of the vegetables on the platter. Serve hot.

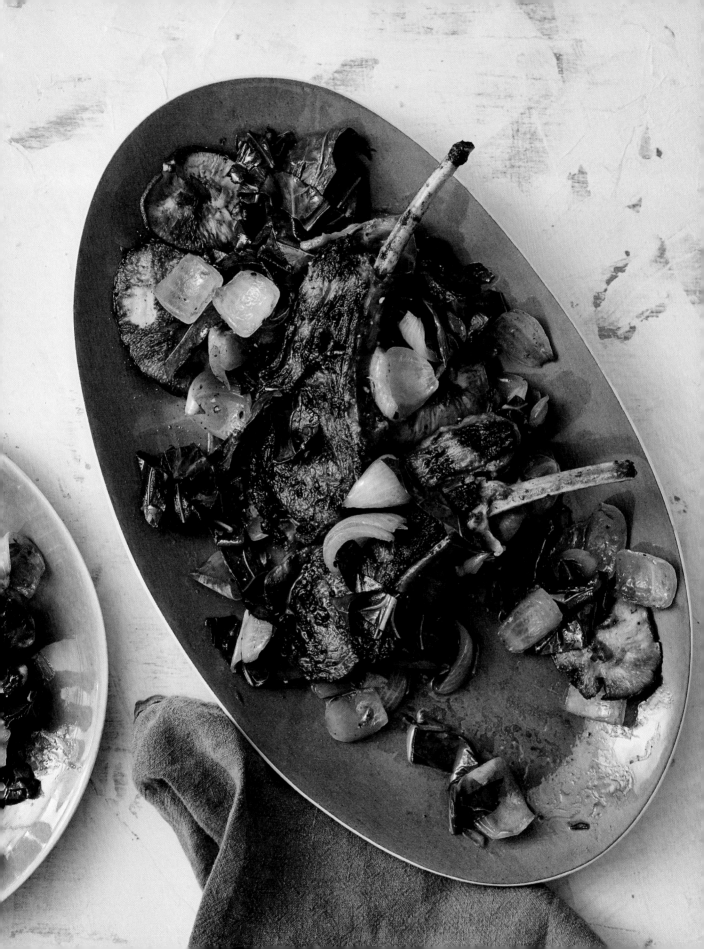

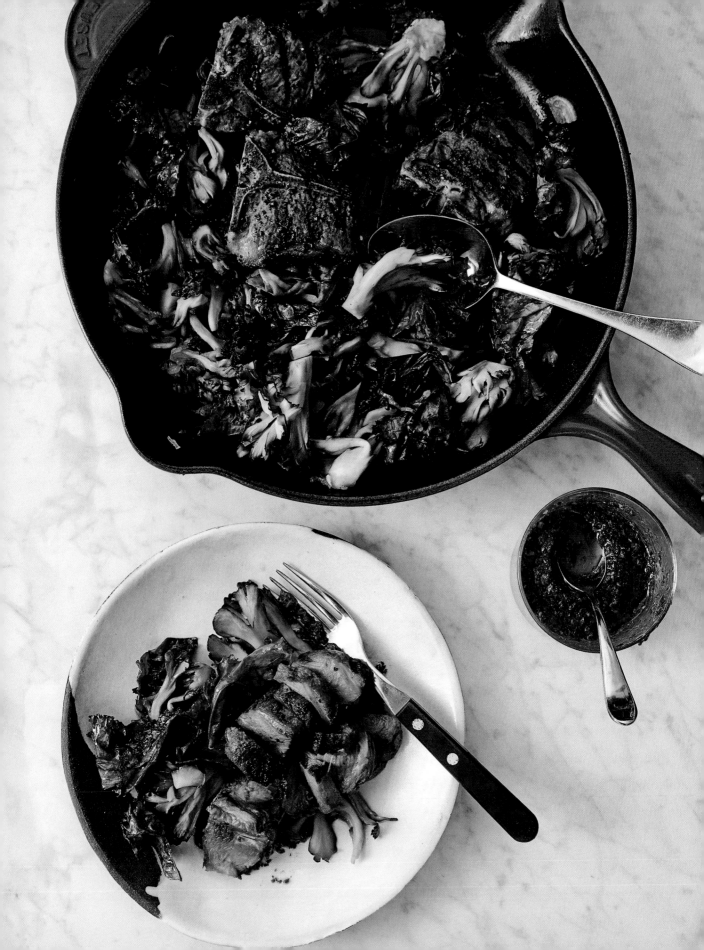

Loin chops have a T-bone running through them, which is what makes them so full flavored. They're best when grilled, as they absorb delicious smokiness. I like to smother these with Sorrel Salsa Verde (page 297) and nestle them in Sautéed Maitake Mushrooms and Mustard Greens (page 104). They're also great on their own, served with a bunch of vegetable dishes.

SERVES
4 TO 8

PERFECTLY GRILLED LAMB LOIN CHOPS

8 (1½- to 2-inch-thick) lamb loin chops (about 3 pounds)

Coarse sea salt and freshly ground black pepper

1 Pat the lamb dry and season with salt and pepper. Let sit at room temperature for 1 hour.

2 Heat a grill to high.

3 Grill the chops, turning every 2 minutes or so, until well browned and beginning to char and a thermometer inserted into the thickest part registers 125°F, 8 to 10 minutes.

4 Let the lamb rest at least 10 minutes before serving.

My mom rarely made burgers for dinner during my childhood—and when she did, she'd serve us goat burgers. I love gamy meat in patties, but I like to make mine extra juicy and packed with the bold tomato heat of harissa. To keep the texture light, I fold in scallions and dandelion greens. If you have ramps on hand, their greens would be great in here, too.

SERVES
4 TO 6

HARISSA SCALLION LAMB PATTIES WITH DANDELION GREENS

I pound ground lamb (77% lean)

I tablespoon mild harissa

¼ cup very thinly sliced scallions

⅓ cup very finely chopped dandelion greens

½ garlic clove, grated on a Microplane

Zest of ½ lemon

2 tablespoons extra-virgin olive oil, plus more for cooking

1½ tablespoons coarse sea salt

I seedless cucumber, peeled and very thinly sliced

Cilantro Za'atar Yogurt Sauce (page 291)

Cilantro sprigs

In a large bowl, combine the lamb, harissa, scallions, greens, garlic, lemon zest, olive oil, and salt. Gently mix with your hands until the seasonings are thoroughly incorporated into the meat, then divide evenly into six balls. Gently pat the balls into 1-inch-thick patties, flattening them while pushing in the sides.

Heat a large cast-iron skillet over high heat. Coat the bottom with olive oil, then add as many patties as can fit comfortably without crowding. Cook, turning once, until nicely seared, about 2 minutes per side. A metal cake tester or thin-bladed knife inserted into the center of a patty should be warm to hot. Repeat with the remaining patties.

Top with the cucumber and serve with yogurt sauce and cilantro sprigs.

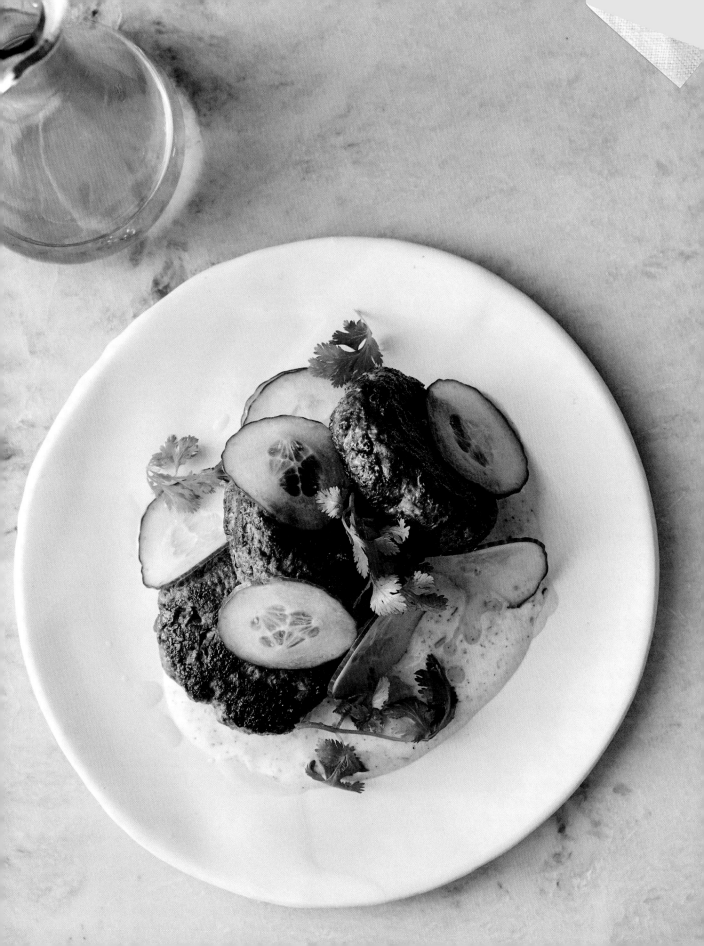

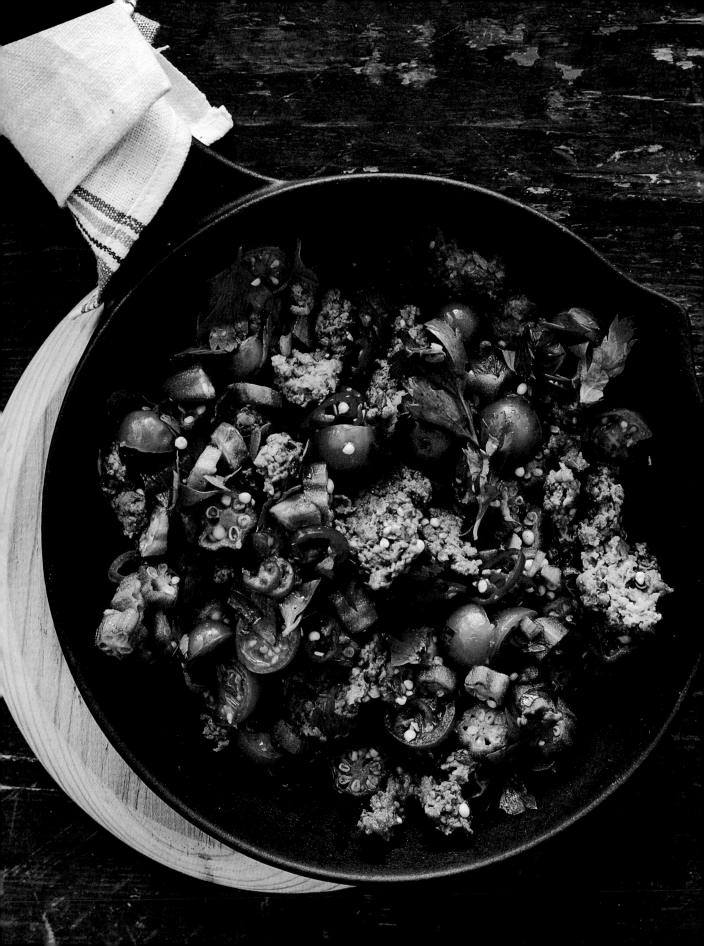

This is sort of like a side dish. You could turn it into an entrée if you slid a fried egg on top. But I created it to showcase the idea of plating food so that the vegetables are as important as the meat. Lamb is just an accent to the okra and tomatoes—albeit a really delicious one—in a Middle Eastern–inspired sauté.

SERVES
2 TO 4

SEARED GROUND LAMB WITH OKRA, CHILES, AND PRESERVED LEMON

2 garlic cloves

4 tablespoons extra-virgin olive oil

¼ preserved lemon, homemade or store-bought, peel only, very thinly sliced

I tablespoon coriander seeds, toasted

I tablespoon sesame seeds

I tablespoon coarse sea salt

8 ounces ground lamb (77% lean)

18 okra pods, cut crosswise into ¼-inch slices

½ cup cherry or grape tomatoes, preferably Sun Golds, halved

½ Fresno chile, seeded if desired, and very thinly sliced

½ cup coarsely chopped fresh herbs, preferably a mix of parsley, mint, and cilantro

Crush and pound the garlic in a mortar with a pestle until flattened. Add 2 tablespoons of the olive oil and mash and stir until the garlic is very finely chopped. Add the preserved lemon peel and pound until the peel is minced. Add the coriander and sesame seeds and pound and stir until they're coarsely crushed. You still want the coriander to keep its fruity pop. Stir in the salt.

RECIPE CONTINUES ▶

OKRA

Okra is super slimy, and that's what makes it special. In fact, that mucilaginous goop is what makes it so high in fiber. As much as I like the slime, I keep okra crisp when I cook it, so it still has some crunch, too.

2 Put the lamb in a bowl and sprinkle the spice mix on top. Mix with your hands until the spices are evenly incorporated into the meat.

3 Heat a large cast-iron skillet over high heat. Add the remaining 2 tablespoons oil and swirl to coat the bottom of the skillet. Add the lamb by dropping it into the pan in bits with your fingers. Spread the meat in a single layer and cook, without stirring, for 2 minutes. Add the okra and cook, stirring often, for 2 minutes. Fold in the tomatoes and remove from the heat.

4 Scatter the chile and herbs on top and serve hot.

TECHNIQUE TIP: Spice mixes ground from whole spices taste so much better when done in a mortar and pestle. Through the pounding, you're forcing ingredients together rather than just blitzing them up in a food processor. Of course, you can use a machine, but go for the old-school option if you can.

Ground milk-soaked almonds take the place of bread crumbs in these herbaceous meatballs, making them richer and more flavorful than classic meatballs. You can enjoy them simply fried, smother them with tomato sauce, or simmer them into stew (see page 236). This recipe makes a big batch, so you can save leftovers to enjoy throughout the week.

SERVES 8 TO 12

SPICED ALMOND LAMB MEATBALLS

2 cups whole milk

1 cup raw almonds

2½ pounds ground lamb (77% lean)

½ cup chopped fresh herbs, preferably a mix of mint, oregano, rosemary, parsley, and thyme

2 garlic cloves, minced

1 tablespoon dry red wine

1 teaspoon cayenne pepper

1 teaspoon ground coriander

1 teaspoon ground cumin

1 teaspoon ground fennel seed

2 large eggs, lightly beaten

2 tablespoons coarse sea salt

½ teaspoon freshly ground black pepper

Extra-virgin olive oil

Combine the milk and almonds in a small bowl and let soak for 30 minutes. Drain the almonds and pulse in a food processor or blender until finely ground. Transfer to a bowl and add the lamb, herbs, garlic, wine, cayenne, coriander, cumin, fennel, eggs, salt, and pepper. Mix with your hands until everything is thoroughly and evenly incorporated. Dampen your hands and shape the mixture into 1-inch-round meatballs.

Heat a large cast-iron skillet over medium-high heat. Generously coat the bottom of the skillet with olive oil. When the oil is hot, add as many meatballs as you can without crowding the skillet, spacing them at least 1 inch apart.

Cook, turning often to evenly brown, until well seared, 3 to 5 minutes. Transfer to paper towels to drain. Serve hot.

This is the ultimate cold-weather meal. Herb-scented broth packed with vegetables, meatballs, and quinoa will warm you up with loads of fiber, protein, and antioxidants. This makes enough to feed a crowd or to keep you ready for a week or more of comforting stew meals.

LAMB MEATBALL STEW WITH QUINOA, BABY CARROTS, SUGAR SNAP PEAS, AND HERBS

2 tablespoons extra-virgin olive oil, plus more for serving

2 carrots, diced

4 cipollini onions, peeled

I cup king oyster mushrooms, cut into I-inch pieces

I fennel bulb, cut into I-inch wedges

2 garlic cloves, sliced

I cup dry white wine

6 cups Chicken Stock (page 139) or store-bought unsalted chicken broth

2 bay leaves

2 thyme sprigs

I rosemary sprig

Coarse sea salt and freshly ground black pepper

I cup red quinoa, rinsed under cold running water and drained

Spiced Almond Lamb Meatballs (page 235)

I jalapeño, thinly sliced

2 cups sugar snap peas, halved

I cup I-inch pieces radicchio

Fresh dill, cilantro, basil, fennel fronds, and mint leaves, chopped

In a large Dutch oven or saucepot, heat the olive oil over medium-high heat. Add the carrots, onions, mushrooms, and fennel and cook, stirring often, for 3 minutes. Add the garlic and cook, stirring, for 1 minute. Add the wine and cook until the alcohol burns off. Add the stock, bay leaves, thyme, and rosemary and bring to a boil. Reduce the heat to maintain a steady simmer. Season with salt and pepper. Add the quinoa and simmer until it's just tender, about 15 minutes.

Add the meatballs, jalapeño, sugar snap peas, and radicchio. Simmer until the vegetables are barely tender but still vibrant, about 3 minutes. Discard the bay leaves. Divide the soup among bowls. Drizzle with oil and sprinkle with herbs.

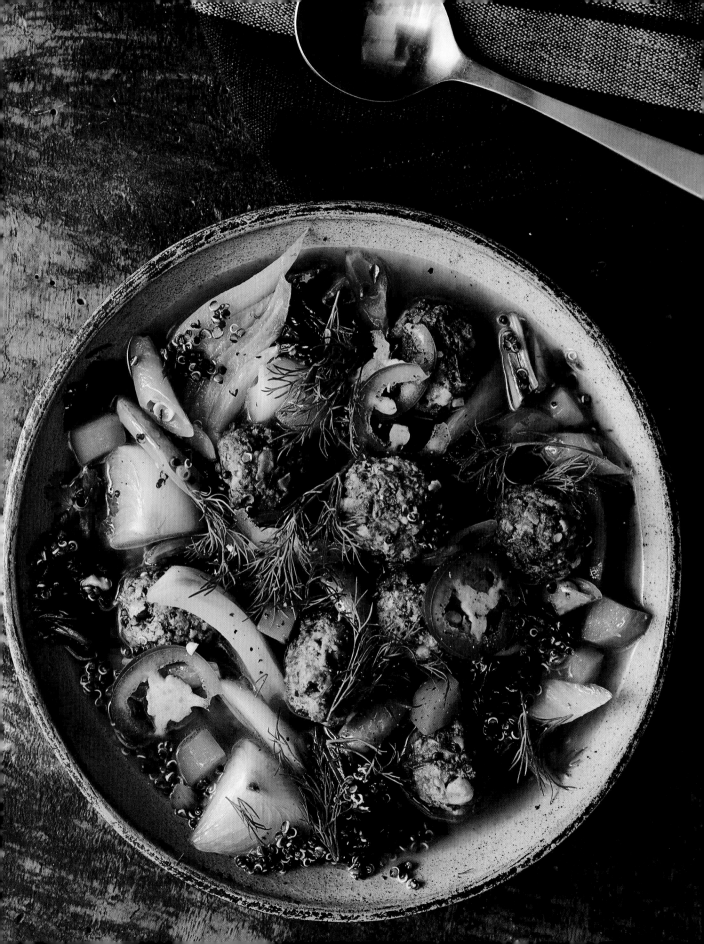

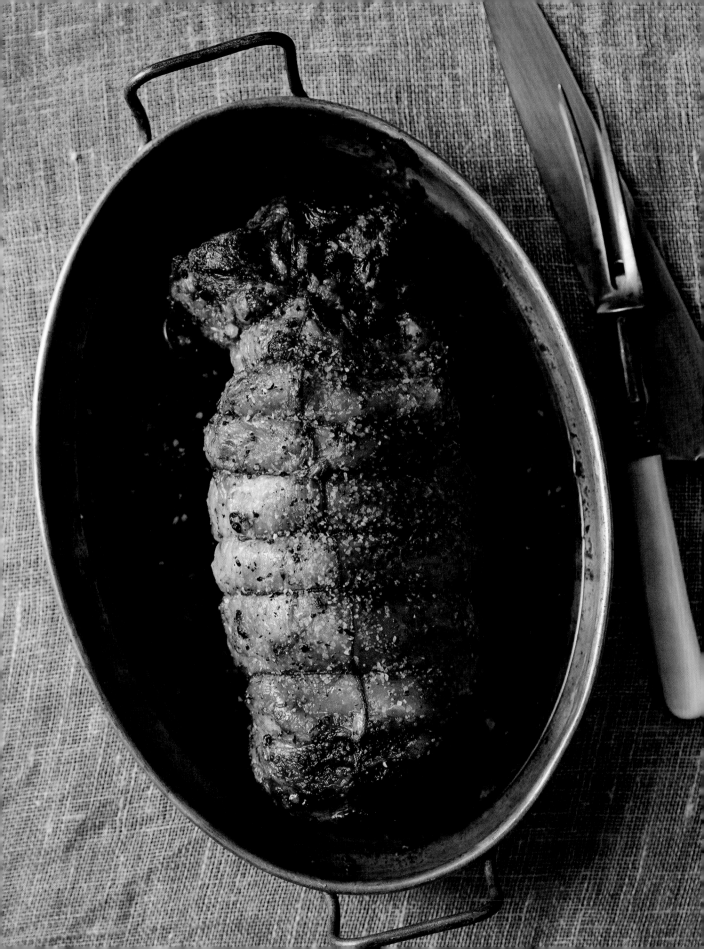

If you're looking for an impressive party dish, you've found it. Savory olives and anchovies rolled into lamb accentuate the meat's big flavors. You can roll and tie the lamb a day or two before roasting it. Carve the spiraled slices in front of your guests and serve with sautéed mustard greens (page 103) or braised kale. To round out the meal, add some grilled leeks, pan-roasted Brussels sprouts (page 127), or squash (page 119).

SERVES 8

ROASTED LEG OF LAMB ROLLED WITH ANCHOVIES, OLIVES, AND HERBS

I shallot, chopped

2 garlic cloves, chopped

½ cup pine nuts

½ cup pitted Kalamata olives

¼ cup anchovies

¼ cup finely grated lemon zest

¼ cup fresh mint leaves

¼ cup fresh flat-leaf parsley leaves

2 tablespoons fresh thyme leaves

½ cup extra-virgin olive oil, plus more as needed

Coarse sea salt and freshly ground black pepper

I (3- to 4-pound) butterflied boneless leg of lamb

Preheat the oven to 425°F. Fit a wire rack in a roasting pan.

In a food processor, pulse the shallot, garlic, nuts, olives, anchovies, lemon zest, mint, parsley, and thyme until finely chopped. With the machine running, add the olive oil. Season with salt and pepper.

Open the lamb, season with salt and pepper, and spread the olive mixture all over the butterflied side. Roll up tightly. Tie in 1½-inch intervals with kitchen twine. Drizzle with oil. Place on the prepared rack, seam-side down.

Roast until the lamb is starting to brown, 30 to 40 minutes. Reduce the oven temperature to 325°F. Roast until an instant-read thermometer inserted into the thickest part registers 125°F, 30 to 35 minutes more. Transfer to a cutting board and tent with foil. Let rest for 15 minutes before slicing.

Lamb shanks, braised until falling off the bone, take well to the intense saltiness of fermented black bean sauce. Onion, garlic, and mushrooms both soak up and lend more aromas to this Chinese-inspired dish. You can find all the ingredients in an Asian market or online.

SERVES
4 TO 6

BRAISED LAMB SHANKS IN LETTUCE CUPS

10 dried shiitake mushrooms

3 garlic cloves

1 (3-inch) piece fresh ginger, peeled and chopped

½ cup fermented black bean and garlic sauce

2 tablespoons Chinese five-spice powder

2 tablespoons Chinese black vinegar

2 dried chiles

1 tablespoon sesame oil

5 tablespoons coconut oil

4 lamb shanks

2 onions, thinly sliced

Coarse sea salt and freshly ground black pepper

2 heads Boston or Bibb lettuce, leaves separated

Pickled Carrots and Daikon (page 269)

Cilantro Salsa Verde (page 295)

1 cup cashews, toasted and coarsely chopped

1   Bring 3 cups water to a boil. Put the dried mushrooms in a medium bowl and pour the boiling water over them. Cover and let stand for 45 minutes.

2   Preheat the oven to 375°F.

3   In a food processor, combine the garlic, ginger, black bean sauce, five-spice, vinegar, chiles, sesame oil, and 3 tablespoons of the coconut oil and puree until smooth, scraping the bowl occasionally. With a sharp knife, cut small slits all over the lamb shanks. Thoroughly coat the shanks with the spice mixture, rubbing it into the slits.

4   In a large Dutch oven or other heavy saucepot, heat the remaining 2 tablespoons coconut oil over high heat. When hot, add the lamb shanks. Cook, turning to evenly brown, until well seared on all sides, 10 to 12 minutes.

5   Meanwhile, spread the onions in an even layer in a roasting pan. Drain the mushrooms in a fine-mesh sieve set over a bowl, reserving the soaking liquid, and scatter the mushrooms on top. Add enough of the soaking liquid to cover the onions. Place the seared shanks on top of the onion-mushroom mixture in a single layer, spacing them apart. Cover the pan tightly with aluminum foil.

6   Transfer to the oven and bake until the meat is so tender it's falling off the bones, about 3 hours. Add more of the mushroom soaking liquid if the pan becomes dry while baking.

7   Carefully transfer the shanks to a dish. Strain the liquid in the pan through a fine-mesh sieve into a large, deep skillet; discard the solids. Bring the liquid to a boil and cook until it has reduced by half. Season with salt and pepper.

8   While the liquid boils, pull the meat off the bones; discard the bones. Transfer the meat to the reduced liquid. Remove from the heat and fold gently until the meat is evenly coated.

9   Divide the lamb among the lettuce leaves. Top with the pickled vegetables and drizzle with the salsa verde. Sprinkle with the cashews and serve immediately.

Rosemary has been shown to increase blood circulation to the brain and to contain anti-inflammatory immune system support compounds. Plus, its piney aroma pairs really well with lamb. That's why I use the stems to skewer the meat and eggplant and the leaves to season the duo. On the grill, everything takes on a smoky, fragrant richness.

GRILLED LAMB AND EGGPLANT KABOBS ON ROSEMARY SKEWERS

8 rosemary stems

8 ounces boneless lamb top round or lamb loin, cut into 1-inch cubes

1 Japanese eggplant, trimmed and cut into 1-inch pieces

Coarse sea salt and freshly ground black pepper

1 lemon

Extra-virgin olive oil

Mint and Parsley Salsa Verde (page 296)

1 Heat a grill to medium-high.

2 Strip the leaves off the rosemary stems, leaving only the leaves at the tops. Coarsely chop the plucked leaves.

3 Season the lamb and eggplant all over with salt and pepper. Zest the lemon directly on top and sprinkle with the rosemary. Drizzle with olive oil and toss until evenly coated. Skewer the lamb and eggplant onto the rosemary stems, alternating the pieces.

4 Grill until nicely browned, about 2 minutes per side for medium-rare. Let rest for a few minutes before slicing and serving with the salsa verde.

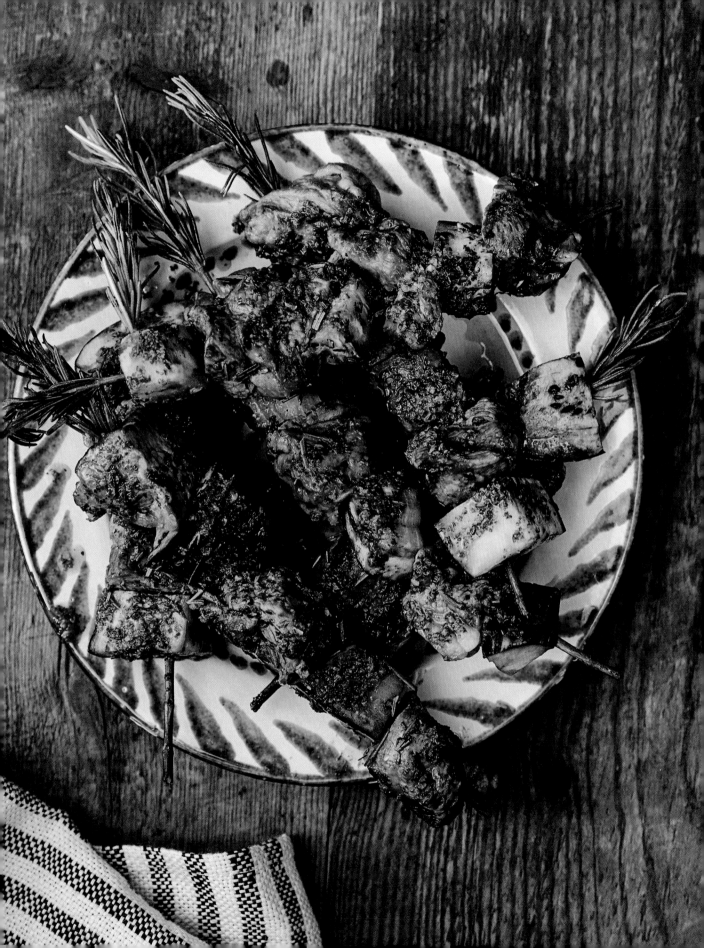

BEEF

You should always buy grass-fed beef. Cows are ruminants. Mother Nature blessed them with complex digestive systems to process grass, and through fermentation in their guts and regurgitation, they can extract nutrients from that fibrous material. A diet of lush grass and hay makes their flesh very high in omega-3 fatty acids.

Feedlot cows are fed corn and soy to make them fat fast with rich marbling that tastes good. Here's how it happens: Cows crammed into filthy, muddy feedlots eating that unnatural grain diet get sick. As a preventative measure, they often are given antibiotics. In fact, industrial farmers figured out a long time ago that by feeding their cattle antibiotics, the cattle got fatter quicker. This may be because there is a direct correlation between cows' gut bacteria and their metabolism. In this unhappy and unhealthy environment, cattle often become aggressive and are prone to goring one another. The stress of this unnatural existence and diet makes them fat and unhealthy. Their flesh ends up being too high in omega-6 relative to omega-3 fatty acids. Omega-6 in and of itself isn't a bad thing, but everything else in a carb-based diet, such as starch, sugar, and commercial oil, is high in omega-6, too.

Cows are monocrop animals that didn't evolve to eat corn and soy. And we didn't evolve to eat cows that eat corn and soy. Eating an unhealthy animal will lead to an unhealthy human. So be sure to buy grass-fed beef from a reputable source, preferably a nearby rancher. Yes, it costs more, but my recipes don't have you eating much of it, so it's worth spending that extra bit for an infinitely better product.

Instead of treating steak like a big solo entrée, I use just a little as part of a vegetable-centric salad. Thin slices made even more savory with a mushroom vinaigrette are super satisfying with a light mix of greens and radishes.

SEARED FLAT-IRON STEAK SALAD WITH RADISHES AND SHIITAKE VINAIGRETTE

I (8-ounce) grass-fed flat-iron steak

Coarse sea salt and freshly ground black pepper

2 tablespoons bacon fat or coconut oil

2 cups mixed greens, such as arugula, baby kale, and mizuna

I cup Chinese green radish or watermelon radish matchsticks

¼ cup red radish matchsticks

½ small red onion, thinly sliced

Shiitake Vinaigrette (recipe follows)

2 tablespoons sesame seeds

Fresh dill and cilantro leaves

Season the steak with salt and pepper. In a large cast-iron skillet, heat the bacon fat over high heat until it begins to smoke. Add the steak and cook, turning once, until well seared, 2 to 3 minutes per side. Transfer to a cutting board and let rest for 5 minutes. Cut the steak into thin slices across the grain.

In a large bowl, combine the greens, radishes, onion, steak and any accumulated juices, and the vinaigrette. Toss until everything is evenly coated. Divide among serving plates and top with the sesame seeds and herbs. Sprinkle with salt and serve immediately.

RECIPE CONTINUES ▶

SHIITAKE VINAIGRETTE MAKES ABOUT 1½ CUPS

I cup dried shiitake mushrooms

2 tablespoons grass-fed unsalted butter

I cup diced rhubarb

½ garlic clove, grated on a Microplane

2 tablespoons white wine vinegar

5 tablespoons extra-virgin olive oil

Coarse sea salt and freshly ground
    black pepper

1   Bring 2 cups water to a boil. Put the dried mushrooms in a small bowl and pour the boiling water over them. Cover and let stand for 25 minutes. Drain well and thinly slice.

2   In a large skillet, melt the butter over medium-high heat. Add the rhubarb, garlic, and drained mushrooms. Cook, stirring often, until softened, 3 to 5 minutes.

3   Add the vinegar and olive oil, stir well, and remove from the heat. Season with salt and pepper. Use warm.

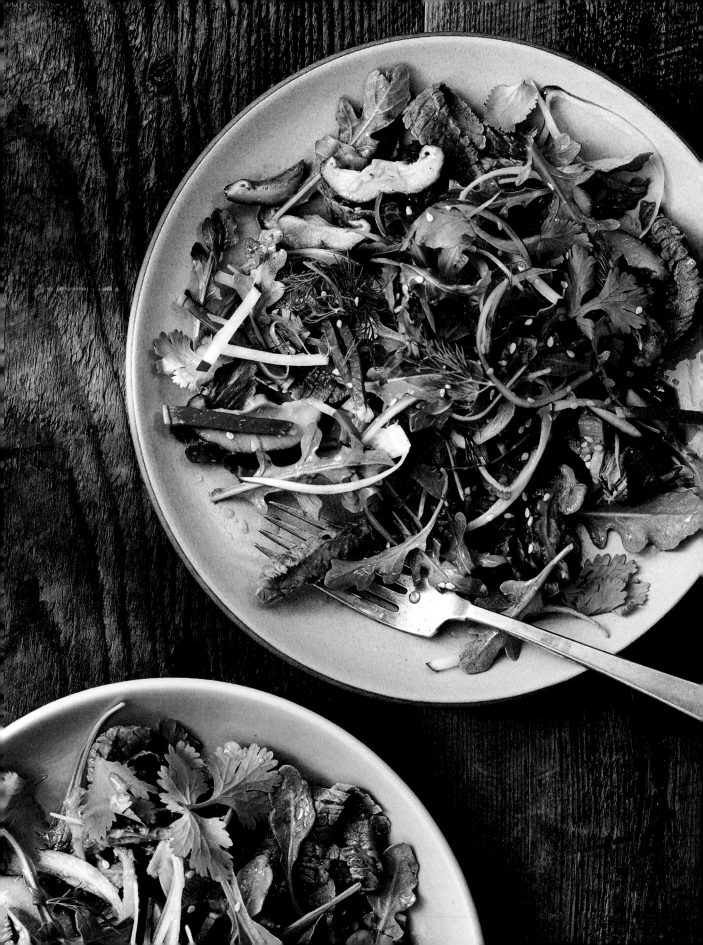

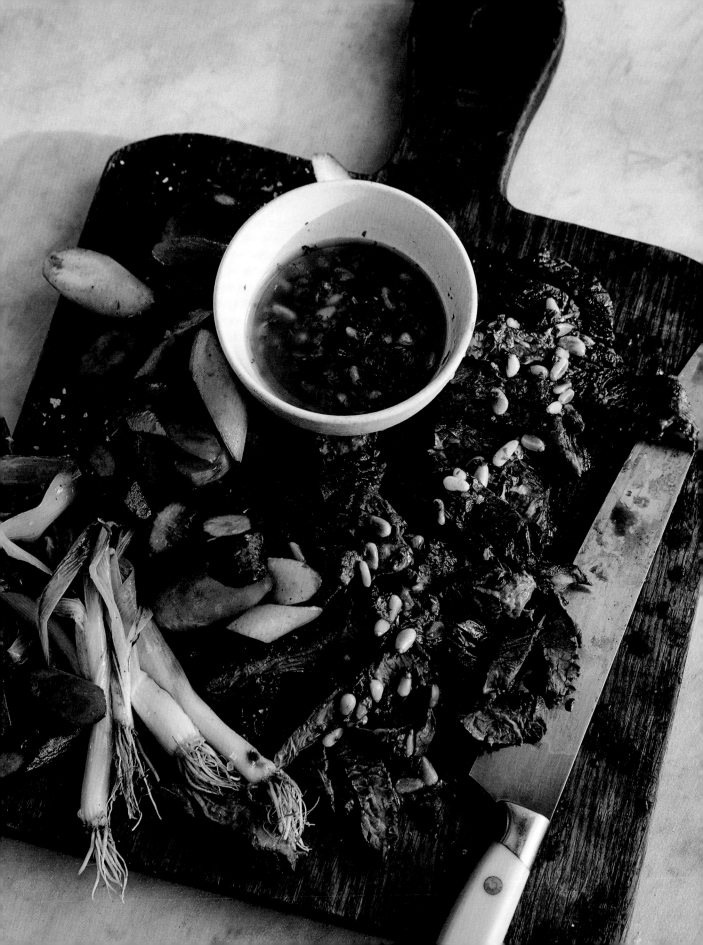

This is a delicious, quick dish that requires only two pans and delivers a perfect balance of healthy protein and vegetables. To get this dinner on the table extra fast, I start by making the chimichurri and setting that aside for the flavors to develop while I cook the steak. While the steak rests, I bang out the vegetables really quickly and then dinner is ready.

SERVES
4 TO 6

GRILLED HANGER STEAK WITH CHIMICHURRI

2 (8-ounce) grass-fed hanger steaks

Coarse sea salt and freshly ground black pepper

I tablespoon coconut oil

2 tablespoons grass-fed unsalted butter

I bunch carrots, cut into I-inch slices at an angle

I bunch spring onions

I teaspoon raw apple cider vinegar

Chimichurri (page 295)

1   Season the steaks generously with salt and pepper. In a large, heavy skillet, heat the coconut oil over high heat. Add the steaks and sear, turning once, until browned, about 2 minutes per side for medium-rare. Add 1 tablespoon of the butter and baste the steaks with a spoon for 1 minute. Transfer to paper towel–lined plates and let rest for 5 minutes.

2   While the steak is resting, in a medium skillet, melt the remaining 1 tablespoon butter over medium-high heat. Add the carrots and spring onions and cook, stirring occasionally, until they begin to soften, 3 to 5 minutes. Season with salt and pepper, then drizzle in the vinegar. Cook, stirring, until the vinegar has reduced and glazes the vegetables, about 1 minute. Divide among serving plates.

3   Slice the steak across the grain and place over the vegetables. Generously drizzle the chimichurri on top and serve immediately.

I've been to Morocco only in my mind, but it's delicious there. My mental image of the food is that it's well spiced with sweet elements. To get that balance here, I bring heat with harissa and ginger and sweetness through raisins and onion. The hearty mix is amazing stuffed into spaghetti squash, but it's also tasty simply spooned over quinoa or other vegetables.

SERVES 4 TO 8

SPAGHETTI SQUASH STUFFED WITH GINGER-GARLIC BEEF

8 ounces ground beef (80% lean)

Coarse sea salt

Extra-virgin olive oil

½ onion, cut into ¼-inch dice

2 garlic cloves, very thinly sliced

1 (2-inch) piece fresh ginger, peeled and very finely chopped

¼ cup pine nuts

¼ cup golden raisins

1 tablespoon harissa, plus more to taste

Harissa Roasted Spaghetti Squash (page 111)

Fresh mint leaves

1   Mix the beef with 1 tablespoon salt. Heat a large cast-iron skillet over high heat. Lightly coat the bottom of the skillet with olive oil. When the oil is hot, add the beef and onion. Cook, stirring and breaking the meat up into tiny bits, for 30 seconds, then add the garlic and ginger. Cook, stirring, for 30 seconds, then add the pine nuts. Cook, stirring, for 15 seconds, then add the raisins.

2   Add the harissa and cook, stirring, for 2 minutes. Remove from the heat. The beef should be cooked through, but the onion and garlic should be barely cooked. Transfer to a large bowl and add the squash. Fold gently until evenly mixed. Add more harissa and salt to taste.

3   To serve, you can mound the mixture back into the squash shells or simply transfer to a serving dish. Tear the mint leaves on top and serve immediately.

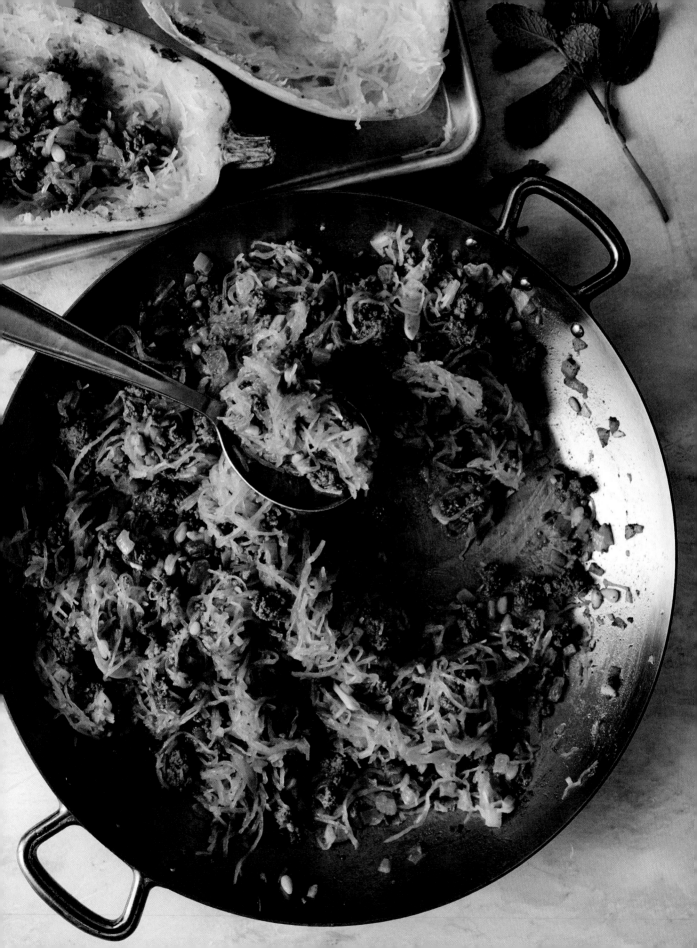

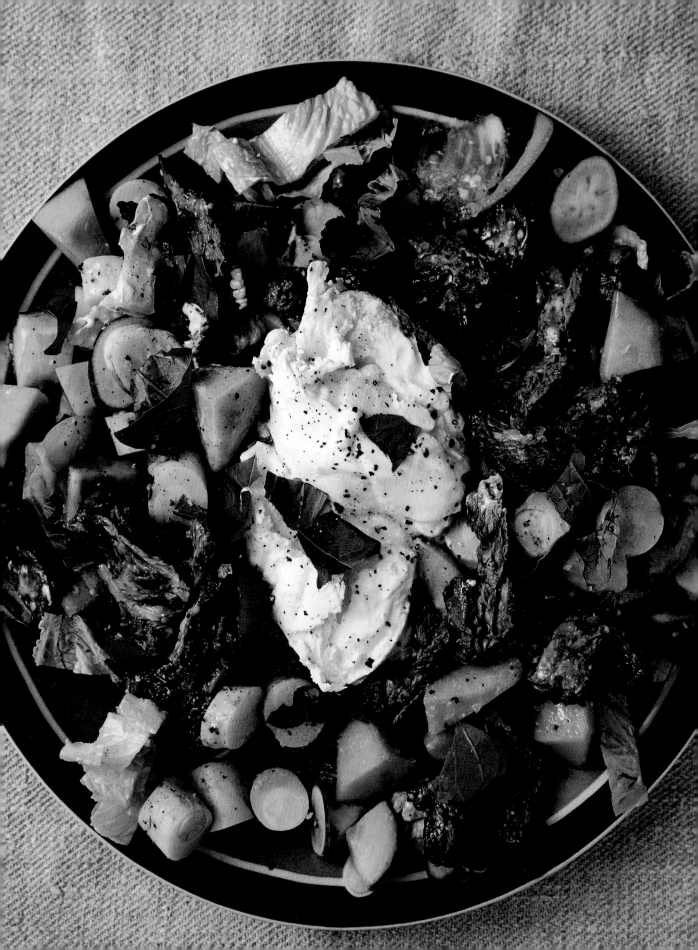

Tomato salad is a steakhouse favorite because it's the perfect pairing of refreshing fruit with smoky meat. To highlight that combo, I throw in juicy cucumber and melon, too, boosting the vitamins in this hearty summer salad.

GRILLED SKIRT STEAK SALAD WITH HEARTS OF PALM, CUCUMBERS, MELON, AND TOMATOES

I pound grass-fed skirt steak

8 ounces fresh or drained canned hearts of palm

Coarse sea salt and freshly ground black pepper

Extra-virgin olive oil

2 pounds mixed heirloom tomatoes, cored and cut into I-inch chunks

I seedless cucumber, cut into I-inch chunks

2 cups fresh melon chunks, preferably Cavaillon melon

I head romaine lettuce, chopped

I shallot, thinly sliced

I cup fresh basil leaves, torn

I small bunch breakfast radishes, thinly sliced

Honey Dijon Vinaigrette (recipe follows)

2 pieces burrata cheese

1 Heat a grill to high.

2 Season the steak and hearts of palm generously with salt and pepper and drizzle with olive oil. Grill the hearts of palm, turning frequently, until nicely charred on the outside and tender on the inside, 3 to 5 minutes. Transfer to a cutting board. Grill the steak until nicely charred, about 3 minutes per side for medium-rare. Transfer to the cutting board. Let the steak rest and the hearts of palm cool.

RECIPE CONTINUES ▶

3   Meanwhile, in a large bowl, combine the tomatoes, cucumber, melon, lettuce, shallot, basil, and radishes. Season with salt and pepper and toss gently to mix. Drizzle the vinaigrette on top and toss until everything is evenly coated.

4   Cut each burrata in half and carefully place each piece, cut-side up, on a serving platter. Sprinkle with salt and pepper and drizzle with oil. Arrange the salad around the burrata.

5   Cut the hearts of palm and the steak into slices, cutting the steak across the grain. Scatter both on top of the salad. Serve immediately.

HONEY DIJON VINAIGRETTE MAKES ABOUT ¾ CUP

I garlic clove, grated on a Microplane

¼ cup champagne vinegar

I teaspoon Dijon mustard

I tablespoon honey

½ cup extra-virgin olive oil, preferably Arbequina

Coarse sea salt and freshly ground black pepper

In a medium bowl, whisk together the garlic, vinegar, mustard, and honey until smooth. While whisking, add the olive oil in a slow, steady stream. Whisk until emulsified. Season with salt and pepper.

PORK

This magical meat has so much flavor. (Bacon has probably broken more vegetarians than any other meat product!) I love pork and find it incredibly satisfying and nourishing when enjoyed in small portions that are integrated with vegetables. If you have a nice pork chop with shaved Brussels sprouts and grilled broccoli raab, it's the perfect meal.

Pork is a naturally lean meat with the exception of specific cuts. The chops and belly have a lot of fat. When those cuts are coming from healthy animals, the fat is actually healthy saturated fat. The shoulder is a great, versatile option that's also very well-marbled—and it's affordable.

As with any ingredient, you want to get the best. At the most basic level, look for pastured, antibiotic-free pork. In a dream scenario you'd know your pig farmers, who are raising a heritage breed and feeding the animals a natural diet of all slop and foraged plants. A good rule of thumb for knowing whether a pig's breed is a heritage one is if it's given a name, such as Berkshire or Mangalitsa.

Historically, we've been told to cook pork to a very high temperature to make up for the risk of pigs that were raised in terrible conditions. Cooking pork beyond well-done is to help mitigate the risk of illness if the meat is tainted. However, when you're using good-quality pork, that's a non-issue. I like pork to have a slightly rosy hue to it and to be nice and juicy. To get that, cook the pork until a meat thermometer inserted in the center registers between 140°F and 145°F, then transfer it to a cutting board and let it rest. The meat will continue to rise in temperature as it sits, and it will stay juicy, too.

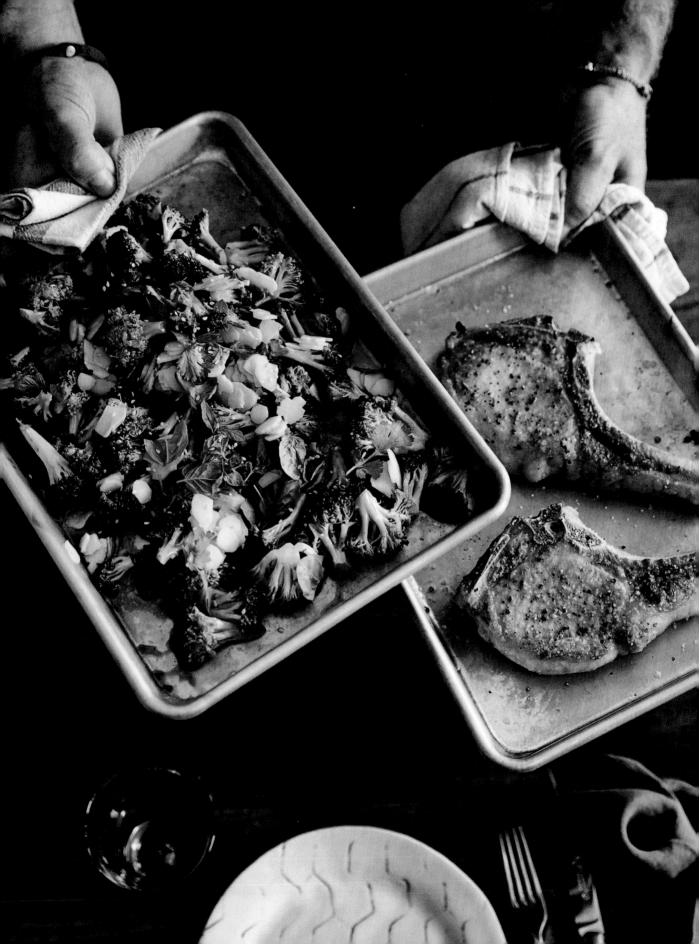

To make really delicious pork chops, start with good pork. My local butcher sells delicious cold-smoked pork chops. They're not cooked, but they have a deep smokiness. If you can't find them, you can use regular pork chops. Ideally get pork chops with their fat caps intact. One common mistake when cooking chops is not getting the oil hot enough before adding the meat. It's okay for the oil to smoke; it'll ensure a deep sear. I like these chops over Broccoli Florets with Gochujang Vinaigrette and Pickled Broccoli Stems (page 114).

SERVES
4 TO 6

SEARED BONE-IN SMOKED PORK CHOPS

2 (1½-inch-thick) bone-in cold-smoked pork chops (about 1 pound each)	Coarse sea salt and freshly ground black pepper	4 tablespoons coconut oil

1 Preheat the oven to 400°F.

2 Heat a large cast-iron skillet over high heat. Very generously season the pork chops on all sides with the salt and pepper. Add the coconut oil and swirl to coat the bottom of the pan. When it's smoking hot, put the chops into the pan, fat cap–side down, and hold them in place with tongs until they're nicely browned, about 1 minute, then carefully lay each chop down on a flat side. Cook until very nicely browned with a deeply colored crust, 1 to 2 minutes per side.

3 Transfer the skillet to the oven and roast for 8 to 10 minutes for medium-rare. Transfer the chops to a cutting board and let rest for 5 to 10 minutes before slicing.

Coppa is the very well-marbled part of the pork shoulder that is used to make coppa, a type of cured meat in Italy. You buy the tied roast, ideally one from a Berkshire pig, from a good butcher. If you can't find coppa, just ask for the fattiest part of the shoulder. To keep the meat moist while roasting, I set it over scallions. I love this with the grape sauce, but it can be served alone with vegetable side dishes, too.

SERVES 4 TO 6

ROAST COPPA PORK SHOULDER

I pound pork shoulder roast, preferably the coppa cut, tied into a tight cylinder with kitchen twine

Coarse sea salt and freshly ground black pepper

I tablespoon rendered leaf lard or extra-virgin olive oil

4 scallions, trimmed

Concord Grape and Ginger Sauce (page 302)

1 Preheat the oven to 400°F.

2 Generously season the pork with salt and pepper. Heat a small cast-iron skillet over high heat. Add the lard and swirl the pan to coat the bottom evenly. When the lard is hot, add the pork. Cook, turning to evenly brown, until well seared on all sides, about 7 minutes.

3 While the pork browns, put the scallions in an even, tight layer on a small rimmed baking pan. Put the pork on top of the scallions and transfer to the oven. Roast until the pork is just cooked through, about 35 minutes. Transfer the pork to a cutting board and let rest for 8 minutes.

4 Snip off the kitchen twine, then cut the pork into ½-inch-thick slices. Divide the pork and scallions among serving plates and drizzle with any accumulated pan juices. Serve hot with the grape sauce.

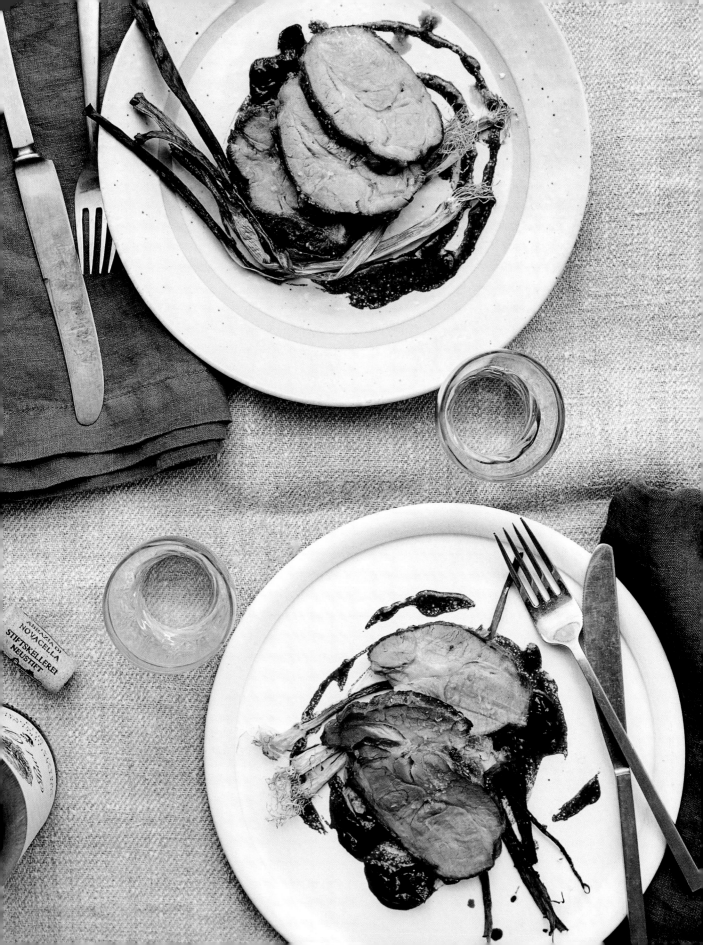

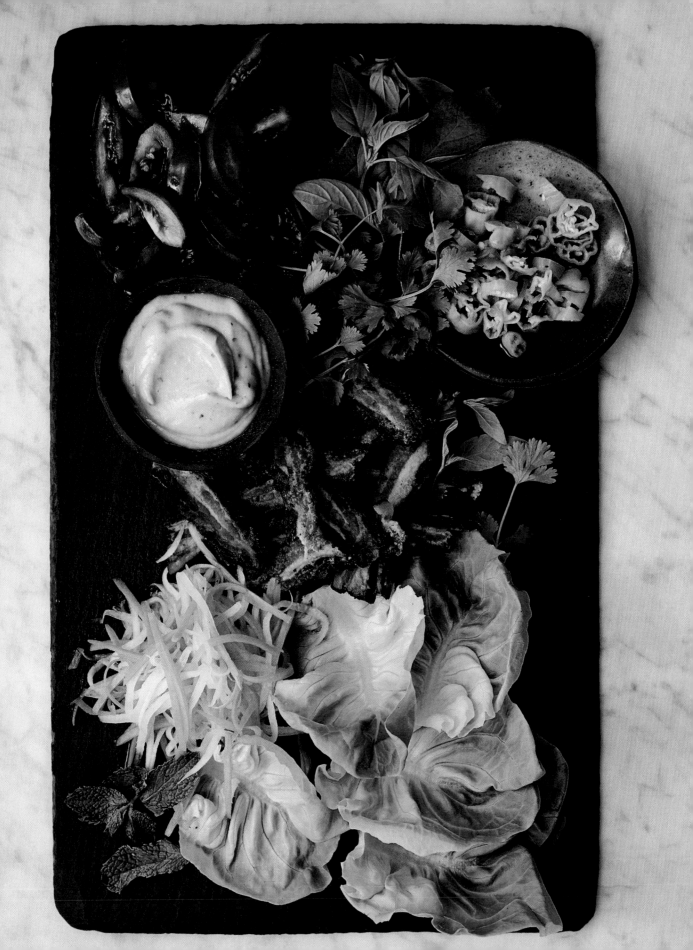

My gluten-free twist on the conventional BLT also has a little Vietnamese flavor pop. This makes only four wraps, but you can easily scale it up to serve a crowd.

SERVES 4

VIETNAMESE BLT WRAPS

4 bacon slices, cooked until crisp

4 large Bibb lettuce leaves

4 tablespoons Avocado Aioli (page 301)

4 cilantro sprigs

4 mint sprigs

4 Thai basil sprigs

4 tablespoons Pickled Carrots and Daikon (page 269)

I heirloom tomato, cored and cut into wedges

2 tablespoons sliced Pickled Peppers (page 270)

1 Put a slice of bacon in each lettuce leaf. Drizzle with the aioli, then top with the herbs, carrot and daikon pickles, tomato wedges, and pickled peppers, in that order.

2 Wrap and enjoy!

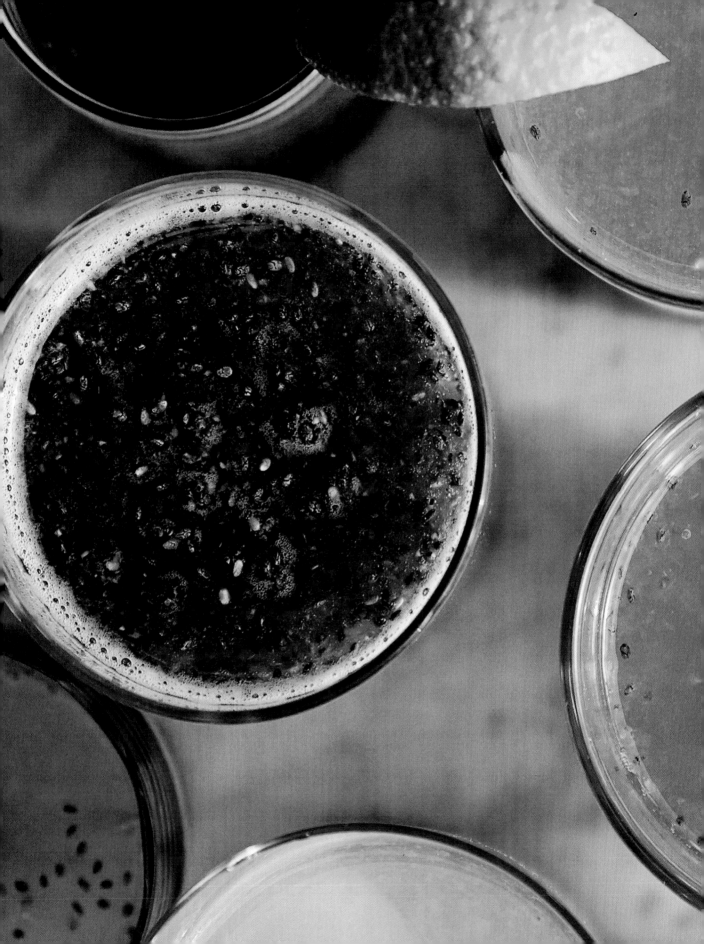

SNACKS & DRINKS

Most days, I have a hearty lunch of soup and salad with some meat among the vegetables, which will keep me full until a light dinner of more vegetables with good fats. I'll then be fine until lunch the next day. Snacking is not something I do very much anymore. When I was not healthy and not eating regular meals, I used to always be in this horrible limbo of not being hungry and being hungry and was much more prone to snacking. In that state, it was so easy to mindlessly pop the most nutrient-deficient and calorie-heavy non-real-foods into my mouth.

I recognize that not everyone can last as long as I do between meals. And there are occasions when I don't have the time to eat a big lunch and light dinner and I do need to snack. When I do, I like having a couple tiny bites of something that's extremely tasty and filling. I typically like crunch because that's satisfying. For grab-and-go snacks, some crudités or a small handful of nuts is enough to keep us from falling into overeating. If I have time, I like to make nori wraps or savor a boiled egg. They're so much more satiating than the junk that surrounds us.

How many times have you told yourself you're just going to have a couple of pretzels and the next thing you know, the bag's half gone? When we have really nutrient-deficient carb-heavy snacks, it's easy to eat too much. Salty, sweet, and crunchy carbs are so easy to binge on, and that unhealthy snack becomes an unhealthy meal.

Just as dangerous are drinks like fruit juices, sodas, and beer. Because they tend to have too much sugar without the benefit of any fiber, the sugar hits our bloodstream fast and hard. Sugary drinks have an extremely deleterious impact on our health if they're part of our regular food rotation.

I'm not saying you should avoid all drinks. That's why when I'm not drinking water, I reach for bright, flavorful homemade mixes that have little to no sugar. When I'm making my own drinks and I'm choosing a sweetener, I'll always go with unrefined options. The resulting mixes are just sweet enough, and a small shot will get your energy going and keep it up for hours.

Seasoning beets before and after cooking accentuates their natural sweetness. I use these in a Marinated Beet Salad (page 79), but also eat them alone or on top of other salads.

MAKES AS MANY AS YOU'D LIKE

ROASTED AND MARINATED BEETS

Beets, preferably a mix of red, gold, and candy-stripe, scrubbed

Coarse sea salt and freshly ground black pepper

Garlic, grated on a Microplane

Thyme sprigs

White wine vinegar

Extra-virgin olive oil

Strips of lemon zest, peeled with a vegetable peeler

Fresh herbs

1 Preheat the oven to 400°F.

2 Put the beets in a bowl, separating the colors into different bowls if using a mix. Sprinkle with salt and pepper and garlic. Toss some thyme on top and drizzle with vinegar. Toss until well coated. Wrap each beet individually in foil and place on a rimmed baking sheet. Roast until tender, about 1 hour. A metal cake tester or paring knife should slide through easily.

3 When cool enough to handle, unwrap, peel, and cut into 1-inch chunks. Transfer to a bowl, separating the colors into different bowls if using a mix.

4 Drizzle with olive oil and top with lemon zest and herbs. Toss until well coated. Enjoy hot, warm, or room temperature. The seasoned beets can be refrigerated for up to 5 days.

This dish is a great swap for chips and guacamole. People are always concerned that guacamole and chips are not a healthy choice. The reality is that the guacamole is really good for you—it's the chips that aren't. This delicious alternative uses crunchy fresh vegetables instead of chips. I get loads of good fats in here by combining avocado with olive oil, yogurt, and pepitas. The toasted seeds also add crunch to the creamy dip. For the crudités, feel free to improvise and use your favorite fresh veggies.

SERVES 4

SUMMER CRUDITÉS WITH AVOCADO DIP

AVOCADO DIP

3 ripe avocados, pitted and peeled

Zest and juice of 3 limes

1 garlic clove, grated on a Microplane

1 tablespoon finely minced serrano chile

¼ cup extra-virgin olive oil

¼ cup plain full-fat Greek yogurt or labne

¼ cup pepitas (hulled pumpkin seeds), toasted

Coarse sea salt

¼ cup chopped fresh cilantro

CRUDITÉS

8 radishes, quartered

1 handful green beans or runner beans, lightly blanched and shocked in ice water (see page 154)

1 small handful asparagus, lightly blanched and shocked in ice water (see page 154)

1 cup cherry tomatoes

2 celery stalks, cut into 3-inch pieces

1 rutabaga, cut into paper-thin slices on a mandoline

1 cup sugar snap peas, lightly blanched and shocked in ice water (see page 154)

1 bunch tricolor carrots, halved lengthwise

1 To make the avocado dip, in a mortar, combine the avocados, lime zest, lime juice, garlic, and chile. Gently pound with the pestle until just mixed. Add the olive oil, yogurt, pepitas, and a pinch of salt and pound and stir until almost smooth but still somewhat chunky. Alternatively, pulse all the ingredients in a food processor. Season with salt.

2 Place crushed ice in a large bowl and nest a small bowl in the middle. Fill the small bowl with the avocado dip and top with the cilantro.

3 Place the crudités around the small bowl, sticking them into the crushed ice. Serve immediately.

Legumes are hard to digest, but vegetables aren't. That's why I make hummus with carrots. They yield a texture that's great for dipping crudités. This dip is elegant enough for a dinner party, but keeps well in the fridge for snacks, too. Serve with crudités, such as cauliflower, radishes, carrots, and cucumbers.

CARROT HUMMUS WITH TURMERIC

2 cups diced carrots

I garlic clove

I teaspoon grated fresh turmeric

2 lemons

½ cup extra-virgin olive oil, plus more for serving

Coarse sea salt and freshly ground black pepper

2 tablespoons hulled, unsalted sunflower seeds, toasted

2 tablespoons sliced fresh mint leaves

Sumac

Crudités, for serving (page 265)

1 Fill a large bowl with ice and water. Bring a small saucepan of water to a boil. Add the carrots and cook until crisp-tender. Drain and immediately transfer to the ice water. When cool, drain again.

2 Transfer the carrots to a food processor and add the garlic, turmeric, and the zest and juice of 1 lemon. Blitz until smooth, adding water 1 tablespoon at a time if the mixture is too thick to blend. You may need to add as much as 4 tablespoons. With the machine running, add the olive oil in a steady stream. Season with salt and pepper.

3 Transfer to a serving bowl and top with the sunflower seeds and mint. Zest the remaining lemon directly on top, drizzle with olive oil, and sprinkle with sumac. Serve with crudités.

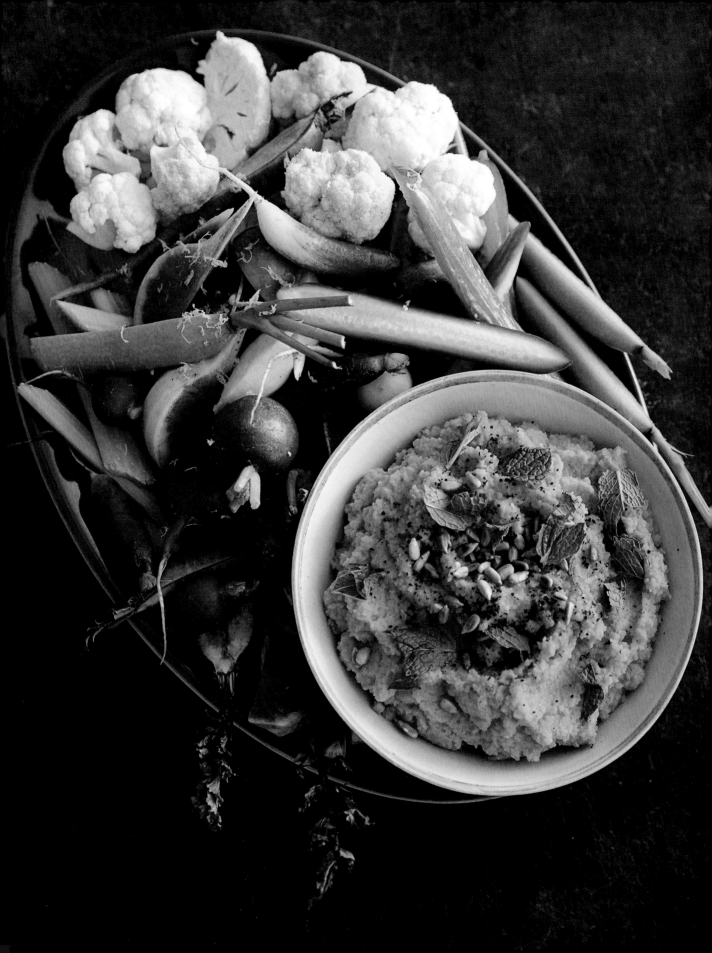

Pickles are so easy to make and so easy to eat. This crunchy homemade version has less sugar and salt than store-bought ones and great probiotic benefits. They're like half-sours with a kick from the chile.

QUICK PICKLED CUCUMBERS

2 large Kirby cucumbers, scrubbed well

2 tablespoons very thinly sliced hot red chile

Coarse sea salt

PICKLING LIQUID

¾ cup raw apple cider vinegar

1 tablespoon raw honey

1 teaspoon coarse sea salt

1 I like to crack the cucumbers, so they're ragged at the edges. To crack them, stick a knife halfway into one cucumber, 1½ inches away from the end. Twist the knife so a 1½-inch chunk of cucumber cracks off. Repeat with the remaining cucumbers.

2 Combine the cucumbers and chile in a large bowl and salt generously. Toss to evenly coat. Transfer to a 1-quart jar or two pint jars.

3 To make the pickling liquid, bring the vinegar, honey, salt, and ½ cup water to a boil in a small saucepan.

4 Pour the hot pickling liquid over the cucumbers. Seal and let sit for at least 20 minutes before using, or refrigerate. The pickles will keep in the refrigerator for up to 1 week.

Chinese and Vietnamese meals often include pickled carrots and daikon. Crunchy and tart, they're a great counterpoint to big savory flavors. I use these in Vietnamese BLT Wraps (page 261) and Braised Lamb Shanks in Lettuce Cups (page 240).

MAKES
ABOUT
2 CUPS

PICKLED CARROTS AND DAIKON

2 cups mixed julienned carrots and daikon

1 tablespoon coarse sea salt

2 cups rice vinegar

¼ cup raw honey

1   In a small bowl, toss the carrots, daikon, and salt. Let sit for 10 minutes. Transfer to a clean kitchen towel and squeeze out all excess moisture. Transfer to a clean pint jar.

2   In a small saucepan, combine the vinegar and honey and bring to a simmer, stirring to dissolve the honey. Remove from the heat and pour over the carrots and daikon. Seal the jar.

3   Let cool to room temperature and use immediately or refrigerate for up to 1 week.

To add a pop of tart heat to any dish, throw on these DIY peppers. I use them in Vietnamese BLT Wraps (page 261), and also enjoy them with vegetables and eggs.

MAKES
ABOUT
I CUP

PICKLED PEPPERS

I cup sliced Anaheim or banana peppers

¾ cup white wine vinegar

¼ cup raw honey

I½ teaspoons coarse sea salt

1 Pack the peppers into a clean half-pint jar.

2 In a small saucepan, combine the vinegar, honey, salt, and ¼ cup water and bring to a simmer, stirring to dissolve the honey and salt. Remove from the heat and pour over the peppers. Seal the jar.

3 Let cool to room temperature and use immediately or refrigerate for up to 1 week.

Sandwiches are the go-to portable lunches of most Americans. I can't deny their convenience, but all that bread and meat drains my energy in the middle of the day. For a lunch that's just as easy to assemble and eat out of hand, I do nori wraps. You can refrigerate the filling in an airtight container, then wrap it in the nori whenever you're ready to eat. If you happen to have Carrot Hummus (page 266) on hand, smear some on the nori, too.

MAKES 1

NORI WRAP WITH GRILLED KING OYSTER MUSHROOMS AND KIMCHI

2 king oyster mushrooms, halved

2 tablespoons extra-virgin olive oil

Coarse sea salt and freshly ground black pepper

¼ cup kimchi

2 tablespoons radish sprouts

1 radish, cut into thin coins

2 tablespoons Carrot-Ginger Vinaigrette (page 86)

1 large sheet nori

2 cilantro sprigs

1 Heat a grill to medium-high or heat a grill pan over medium-high heat.

2 Toss the mushroom halves with the olive oil and season with salt and pepper. Grill, turning occasionally, until browned and tender. Transfer to a cutting board and cut into slices.

3 Place the mushrooms in a medium bowl and toss in the kimchi, sprouts, radish, and vinaigrette. Spoon in a line in the center of the nori and top with the cilantro sprigs. Wrap and eat immediately.

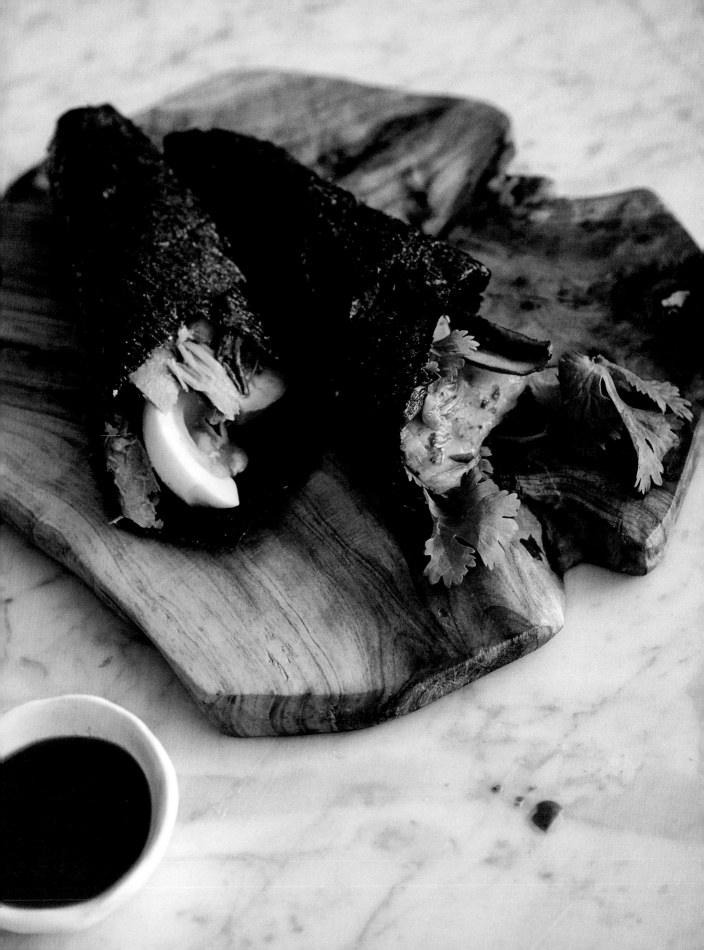

When I need a filling and quick snack or lunch, I pile my favorite staples into nori. It's like a sushi hand roll, but doesn't require the skills of a sushi chef. All the savory ocean umami here—seaweed, anchovies, and tuna—makes the flavor satisfying, and the richness of avocado and egg make it filling.

MAKES AS MANY AS YOU WANT

NORI WRAP WITH AVOCADO, BOILED EGG, ANCHOVIES, AND TUNA WITH HOT SAUCE

All you have to do to make this wrap is fill a nori sheet with a few avocado slices, a quartered Just-Right Boiled Egg (page 306), a fillet or two of anchovy, and flaked chunks of good-quality olive-oil packed tuna. Squirt Sriracha or your favorite hot sauce on top, fold in the sides, and start eating!

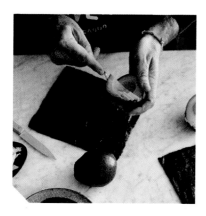
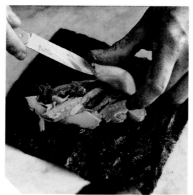
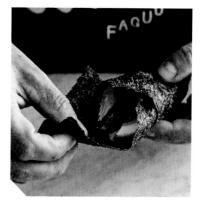

Most store-bought bars are loaded with refined sugar and questionable ingredients. And they often taste stale. I prefer to make my own, which come together in minutes. These are the snacks I pack when I'm going for long bike rides because they provide slow-burning fuel that keeps me going at a steady pace. If you can't find cacao butter, simply substitute coconut oil. I like to store these bars in an airtight container in the freezer. When I want one, I take it out and let it soften for a few minutes before I eat it.

**MAKES
12 BARS**

TROPICAL ENERGY BAR

2 cups unsalted macadamia nuts

2 cups no-sugar-added dried pineapple

1 cup unsweetened dried coconut flakes

2 tablespoons coconut oil

¼ cup cacao butter

1 tablespoon chia seeds

1 teaspoon coarse sea salt

1 Combine all the ingredients in a food processor. Pulse until the mixture resembles a dry cookie dough. If you need to add a little moisture, drizzle in a little cold water.

2 Spread the mixture on a medium rimmed baking sheet lined with plastic wrap. Cover with plastic wrap and press firmly into an even layer.

3 Using a sharp knife, cut into 12 bars. Wrap each individually with waxed paper or plastic wrap. Freeze in an airtight container for up to 3 months.

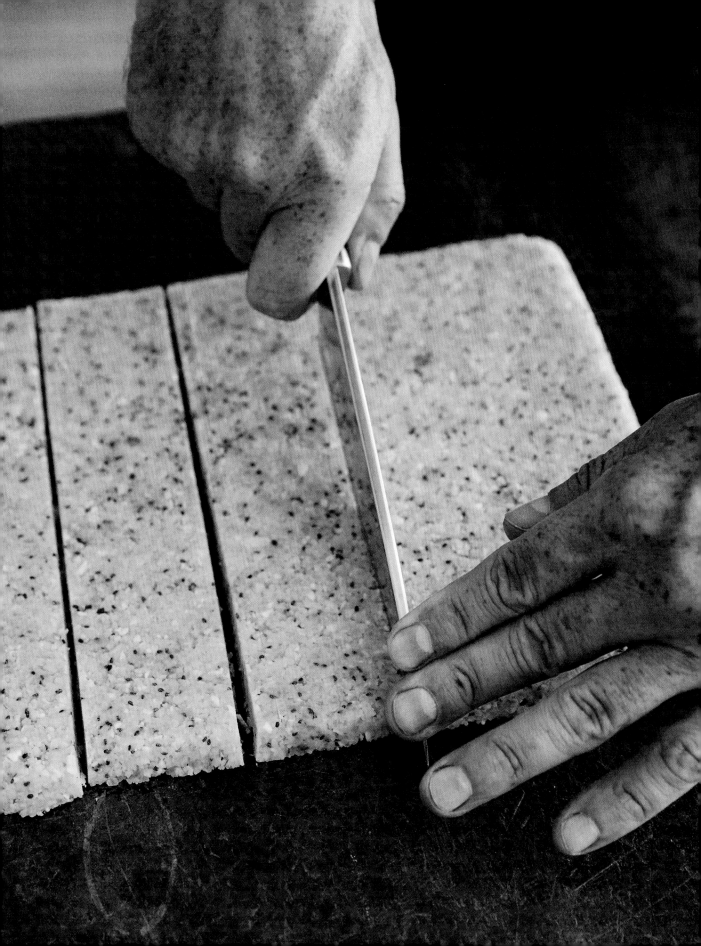

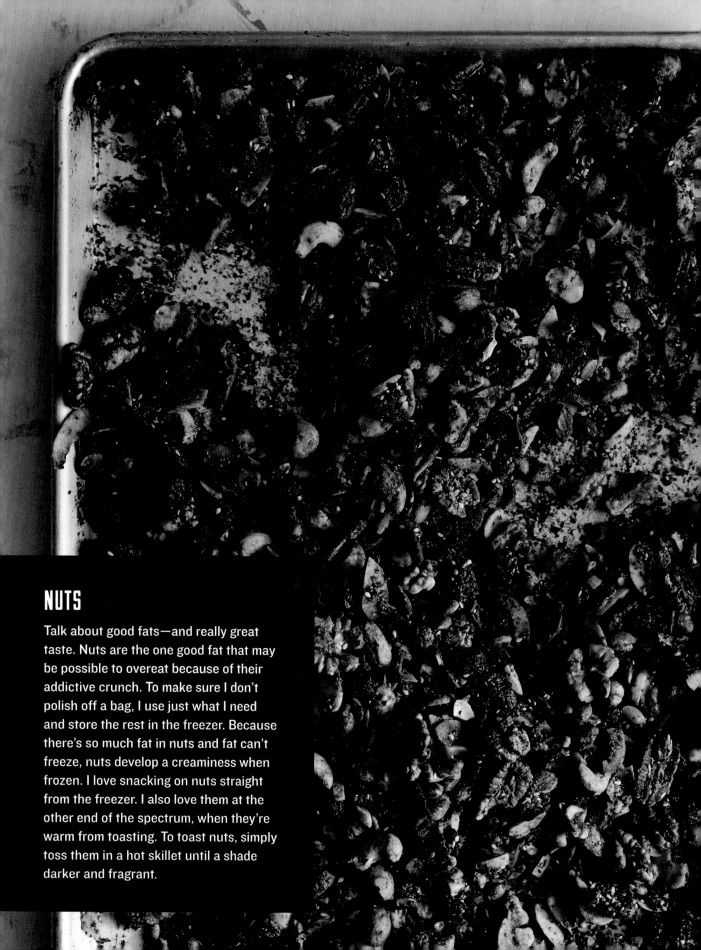

NUTS

Talk about good fats—and really great taste. Nuts are the one good fat that may be possible to overeat because of their addictive crunch. To make sure I don't polish off a bag, I use just what I need and store the rest in the freezer. Because there's so much fat in nuts and fat can't freeze, nuts develop a creaminess when frozen. I love snacking on nuts straight from the freezer. I also love them at the other end of the spectrum, when they're warm from toasting. To toast nuts, simply toss them in a hot skillet until a shade darker and fragrant.

Most granola has loads of oats as filler. My grain-free version does away with the oats and combines all my favorite nuts, seeds, and dried fruits instead. By slowly roasting the mix with maple syrup and coconut oil, I give it a super-tasty crunch that lasts for weeks. (But mine is usually completely gone long before that!)

**MAKES
ABOUT
7 CUPS**

SIMPLY THE BEST GRANOLA

¾ cup pecans

¾ cup walnuts

½ cup slivered almonds

½ cup sliced almonds

½ cup pepitas (hulled pumpkin seeds)

½ cup cashews

¼ cup flaxseeds

¼ cup flaxseed meal

¼ cup sesame seeds

¾ cup unsweetened dried coconut flakes

5 dates, pitted and chopped

¼ cup chia seeds

¼ cup dried tart cherries

½ cup macadamia nuts

¼ cup dried mulberries

½ cup shelled pistachios

¼ cup coconut oil, warmed until liquid

⅔ cup pure maple syrup

1½ teaspoons Jacobsen flake finishing sea salt, slightly crushed

1 teaspoon ground cinnamon

1 Preheat the oven to 325°F. Line a rimmed baking sheet with parchment paper.

2 Combine all the ingredients in a very large bowl and fold gently until everything is evenly coated. Spread in an even layer in the prepared pan.

3 Bake, stirring every 10 minutes or so, until deep golden brown, about 40 minutes.

4 Let cool completely in the pan on a wire rack. The nuts will crisp as they cool. The granola can be stored in an airtight container at room temperature for up to 3 weeks.

Switchel is a maple syrup, ginger, and vinegar–based drink that I like to think of as a Vermonter's Gatorade. It's popular in my home state and is a great way to replenish electrolytes and improve gut health. I make mine with Bragg apple cider vinegar and Vermont syrup (of course!). My buddy Ted King, a retired pro cyclist and founder of UnTapped Maple, uses packets of the most amazing Vermont maple syrup as portable food on the bike. It's rich with manganese, zinc, and potassium, and a natural source of antioxidants, making it great for muscle recovery!

MAKES ABOUT 10 CUPS

SWITCHEL

I cup chopped peeled fresh ginger

¾ cup pure maple syrup, preferably UnTapped Maple

I tablespoon sea salt

¾ cup raw apple cider vinegar

Zest and juice of I lemon

I tablespoon magnesium powder (optional)

1 Put the ginger in a blender with a few tablespoons water. Blitz until very finely chopped, adding more water if needed to get the blender going and scraping the bowl occasionally. Transfer to a small saucepan and add 2 cups water. Bring to a boil, then remove from the heat and stir in the maple syrup and salt until both dissolve. Let steep for 15 to 20 minutes.

2 Transfer to a large pitcher or jar. Stir in the vinegar, lemon zest, lemon juice, magnesium powder (if using), and 8 cups water.

3 Refrigerate until very cold. Stir or shake before serving.

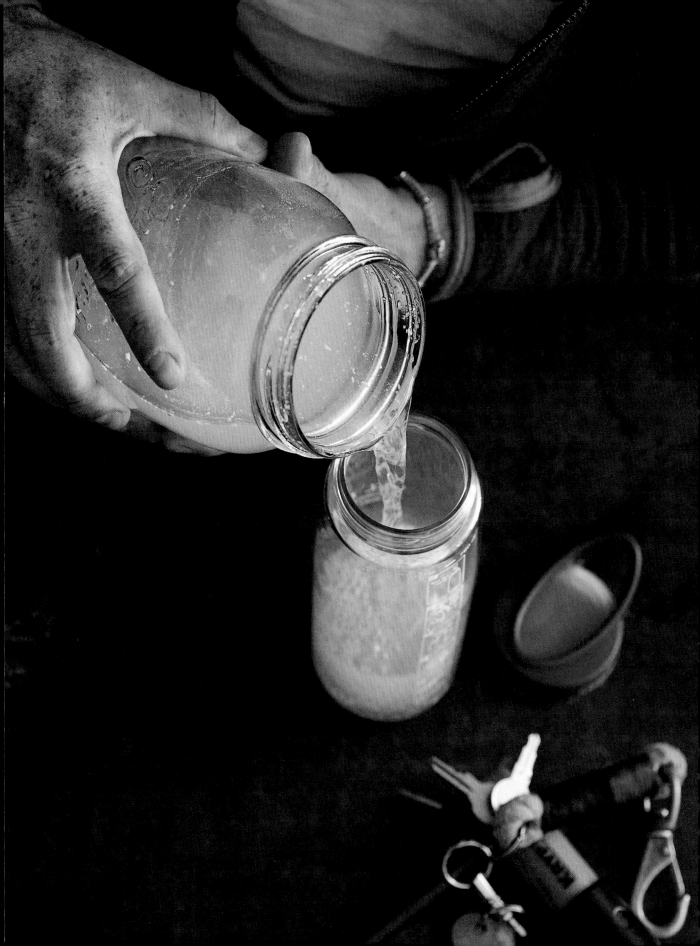

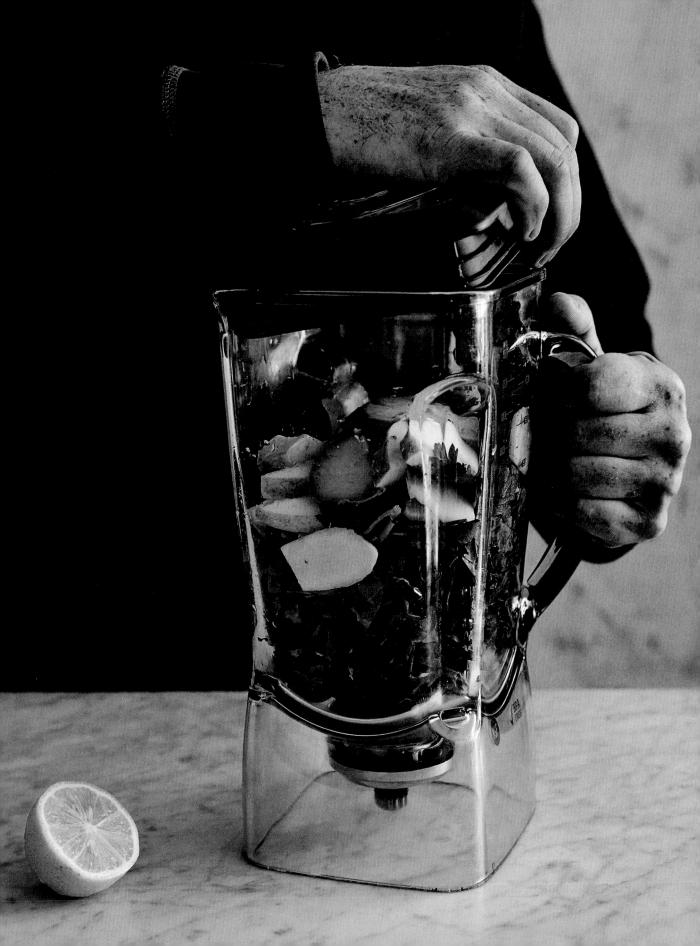

Smoothies combine all the vegetables normally found in green juice, but keep their fiber and, frankly, their flavor intact. This is my favorite green version.

SMOOTHIE WITH KALE, AVOCADO, AND PEAR

I cup fresh flat-leaf parsley

I cup chopped kale

I (I-inch) piece fresh ginger, peeled

I ripe pear, cored

Juice of 2 lemons

I tablespoon raw honey

I avocado, pitted and peeled

In a blender, combine the parsley, kale, ginger, pear, lemon juice, honey, and 2 cups ice water. Puree on high speed until smooth. Add the avocado and blend on medium speed until creamy. If it's too thick for your taste, blend in more ice water.

This is a bright, fresh, and vibrant way to start the day with good fats, micronutrients, and antioxidants all in one glass. Just note that you'll need to let the chia seeds soak overnight first.

MAKES 1

BLUEBERRY CHIA TONIC

I tablespoon chia seeds

¼ cup fresh or frozen blueberries

I teaspoon chopped peeled
fresh ginger

Pinch of sea salt

1 Stir the chia seeds with 1 cup water in a pint-size glass jar. Cover and refrigerate overnight.

2 In the morning, in a blender or food processor, combine the blueberries, ginger, and salt and pulse until smooth. Add to the jar with the soaked chia seeds and screw on the lid tightly. Shake vigorously and drink or pop back in the fridge for later. Shake again before drinking.

282   REAL FOOD HEALS

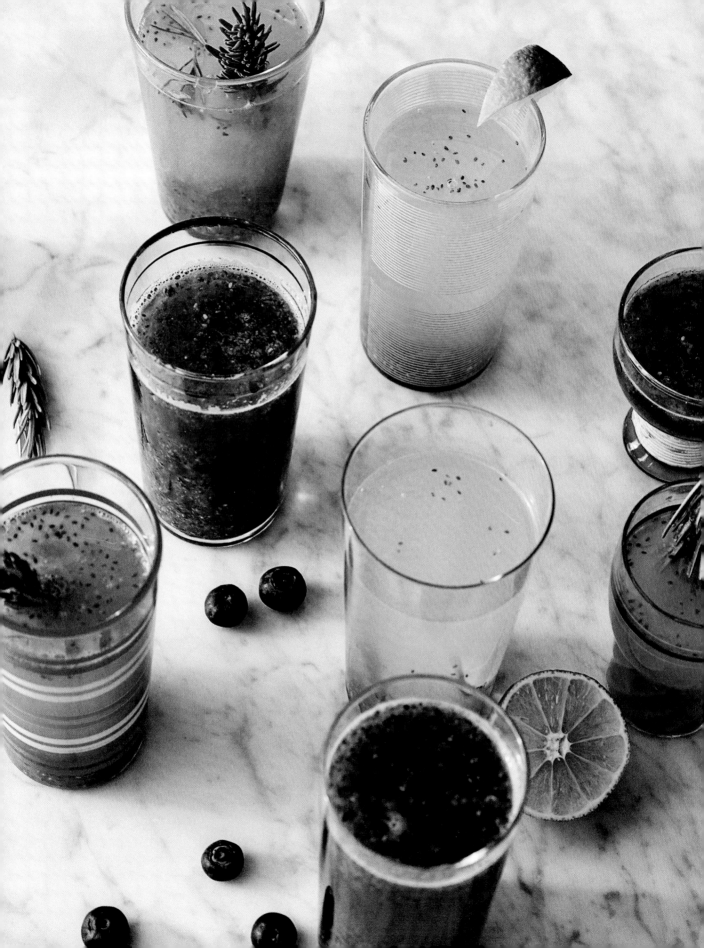

Three ingredients equal an incredibly refreshing drink. You can adjust the lime juice and maple syrup balance to your taste after mixing with the chia seeds and water.

LIME AND MAPLE CHIA TONIC

| I tablespoon chia seeds | Juice of 2 limes | I tablespoon pure maple syrup |

1 Mix the chia seeds, lime juice, maple syrup, and 2 cups water in a glass jar. Seal the jar and refrigerate for at least 2 hours and up to overnight, shaking occasionally.

2 Shake again before drinking.

Grapefruit and rosemary are easy to find in winter and taste terrific together. I love how vibrant this feels on cold, gray days.

ROSEMARY AND GRAPEFRUIT CHIA TONIC

| 1 tablespoon chia seeds | Juice of 1 grapefruit | 1 rosemary sprig |

1   Mix the chia seeds, grapefruit juice, rosemary, and 2 cups water in a glass jar. Seal the jar and refrigerate for at least 2 hours and up to overnight, shaking occasionally.

2   Discard the rosemary. Shake again before drinking.

ROSEMARY

This pine-scented herb has been shown to increase blood circulation to the brain and contains anti-inflammatory immune system–support compounds.

Even though this has no added sugar, it's delicious enough to be dessert. Chia seeds plumped in creamy coconut and almond milk taste almost like tapioca pudding. A really ripe mango delivers luscious tropical sweetness to the mix.

CHIA PUDDING WITH PUREED MANGO

½ cup chia seeds

I cup unsweetened almond milk

I cup unsweetened coconut milk

2 cups diced mango

¼ cup unsweetened dried coconut flakes, toasted

Jacobsen flake finishing sea salt

1 In a large bowl, stir together the chia seeds, almond milk, and coconut milk. Let stand, stirring occasionally, until thickened, about 10 minutes.

2 Meanwhile, in a blender or food processor, puree the mango until smooth. Divide among four small glass jars. Pour the chia mixture on top of the mango puree. Seal the jars and refrigerate until cold.

3 When ready to serve, sprinkle with the coconut and a small pinch of salt.

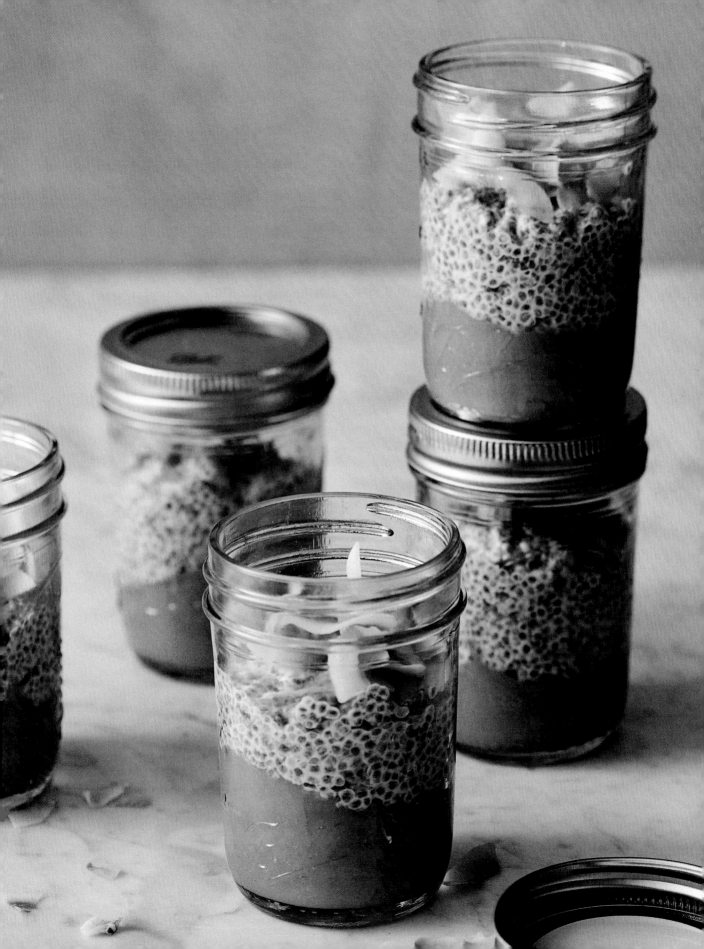

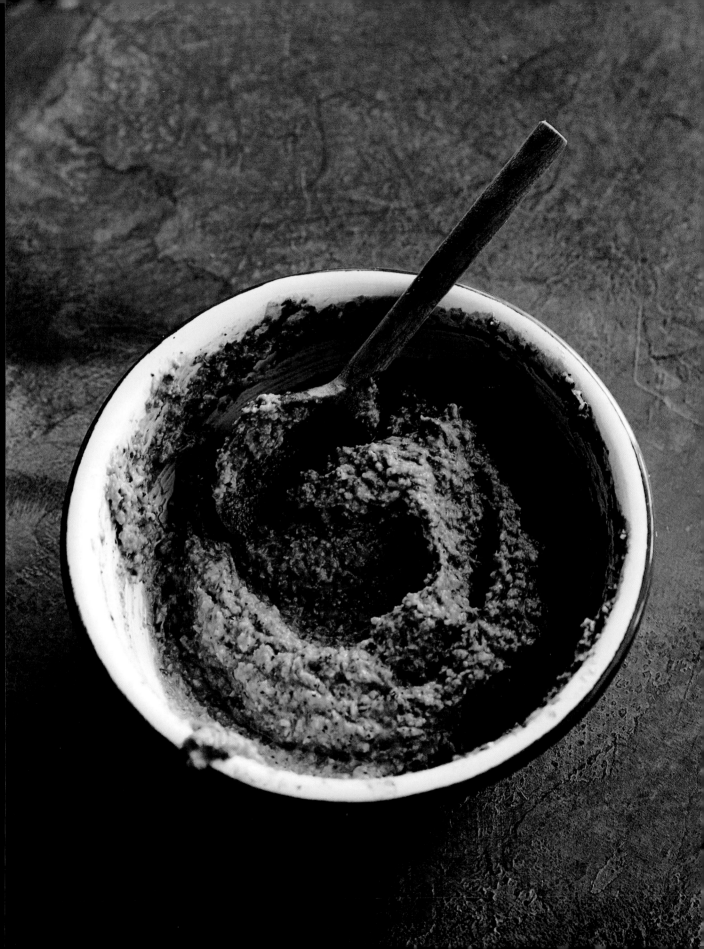

SAUCES & STAPLES

Setting yourself up for success means having a well-stocked pantry. Surround yourself with great ingredients. It's hard to make bad decisions when you don't have bad options. When you have good raw materials to work with, it opens up the possibilities for making great food. Sometimes, that means making extra chimichurri for dinner tonight so you can save some for a salad dressing for lunch the next day.

I also love the notion of using unconventional sauces for vegetables, meats, and fish. Whether that means chopped herbs with dried fruit and nuts or stone fruit in a vinaigrette or chunky salsa, a surprising sauce can give a dynamic layer to a dish. It can create a point of contrast or complement flavors in unexpected ways.

Most people don't think twice about ordering poached eggs with hollandaise at a restaurant brunch, but the thought of saucing fried eggs at home is a leap of creativity. I encourage that creativity by making sure the herb pestos and salsa verdes intended for dinner yield leftovers, so you can have an incredibly exciting and inspiring addition to breakfast eggs.

Smooth and silky, this mint sauce is for drizzling over Marinated Spice Grilled Carrots (page 124). It is also good as a dressing for hearty vegetables or as a sauce for grilled lamb.

MAKES ABOUT 1½ CUPS

MINT YOGURT SAUCE

1 cup plain full-fat yogurt

1 garlic clove

Zest and juice of 1 lemon

1 cup fresh mint leaves

½ cup extra-virgin olive oil

Coarse sea salt and freshly ground black pepper

In a blender, combine the yogurt, garlic, lemon zest and juice, and mint and puree until smooth and pale green. Pour into a medium bowl and whisk in the olive oil until smooth. Season with salt and pepper.

Fine bits of herbs lace this sauce, which I dollop onto Chilled Pea Soup (page 155). You can try it on other chilled soups, too, or use it as a dip for vegetables.

MAKES ABOUT 1¼ CUPS

HERBED YOGURT

1 cup plain full-fat yogurt

1 garlic clove, grated on a Microplane

Zest and juice of 1 lemon

¼ cup minced fresh mint leaves

¼ cup minced fresh flat-leaf parsley leaves

1 tablespoon fresh thyme leaves

¼ cup extra-virgin olive oil

Coarse sea salt and freshly ground black pepper

In a medium bowl, combine the yogurt, garlic, lemon zest and juice, mint, parsley, thyme, and olive oil. Stir until well mixed and season with salt and pepper.

Juicy, tart pomegranate seeds and the floral zing of pink peppercorns punctuate this lemony sauce. I spoon it over Ras el Hanout Roasted Kabocha Squash (page 119). It's also great over roasted root vegetables.

MAKES ABOUT
1¼ CUPS

POMEGRANATE YOGURT SAUCE

I cup plain full-fat yogurt

½ garlic clove, grated on a Microplane

¼ cup extra-virgin olive oil, preferably Arbequina

Zest and juice of I lemon

1½ teaspoons freshly ground pink peppercorns

Seeds of ½ pomegranate

2 tablespoons chopped fresh mint

Coarse sea salt

In a medium bowl, combine the yogurt, garlic, oil, lemon zest and juice, pink pepper, pomegranate seeds, and mint and stir until very well mixed. Season with salt.

Just a pinch of za'atar deepens this cilantro yogurt sauce. I serve it with Harissa Scallion Lamb Patties with Dandelion Greens (page 230). It'd be just as welcome on any other lamb dish.

MAKES ABOUT
⅔ CUP

CILANTRO ZA'ATAR YOGURT SAUCE

½ cup plain full-fat yogurt or labne

½ lemon

½ lime

2 tablespoons finely chopped fresh cilantro

2 tablespoons extra-virgin olive oil

¼ teaspoon za'atar

Coarse sea salt and freshly ground black pepper

Place the yogurt in a small bowl. Zest the lemon and lime directly over the yogurt. Squeeze in the juice from the lime; reserve the lemon for another use. Add the cilantro, olive oil, and za'atar and stir well. Season with salt and pepper.

Diced cucumbers bring crunch and another level of fresh to this kefir sauce. I drizzle it all over Seared Kefir-Marinated Chicken and Tomato Skewers (page 203). You can use it as a sauce for any grilled meats or spoon it over quinoa.

MAKES ABOUT 2 CUPS

GINGERED CUCUMBER KEFIR RAITA

I cup plain full-fat kefir

½ garlic clove, grated on a Microplane

I tablespoon grated peeled fresh ginger

Zest and juice of I lemon

¼ cup fresh mint, finely chopped

¼ cup fresh cilantro, finely chopped

½ seedless cucumber, peeled and cut into ½-inch dice

2 tablespoons extra-virgin olive oil

¼ teaspoon Espelette pepper or paprika

Coarse sea salt

Combine all the ingredients in a medium bowl and fold together until well mixed. Season with salt. Refrigerate for at least 30 minutes before serving to let the flavors develop.

Keeping the rind on lemon slices adds a delicious bitter edge and full-bodied texture to this parsley pesto. Use it as is to slather on Grilled Zucchini Planks (page 110) or grilled eggplant slices or onions. Or thin it with a little oil and vinegar and use it to dress a purslane salad or other wild greens.

MAKES ABOUT 2 CUPS

CASHEW, ANCHOVY, AND LEMON PESTO

I cup cashews, toasted

2 garlic cloves, chopped

6 paper-thin slices lemon, seeded

I dried guindilla chile or I teaspoon red pepper flakes

2 anchovy fillets

½ cup fresh flat-leaf parsley leaves

I cup extra-virgin olive oil

Coarse sea salt and freshly ground black pepper

In a mortar, combine the cashews, garlic, lemon, chile, anchovies, and parsley. Pound with the pestle until everything is chopped and crushed. Add the olive oil and stir and gently pound until the mixture forms a chunky paste. Season with salt and pepper.

Fresh parsley, mint, and dill mellow the sharp kick of garlic scapes in this pesto, as do pistachios. A generous helping of anchovies in the pesto makes this super savory and ideal for any dish or ingredients that could use a flavor boost. I toss it with Zucchini Noodles (page 100) and mix it into a dressing for Arugula and Cucumber Salad with Prosciutto and Parmesan (page 54). You could serve it with grilled swordfish or sautéed summer squash, too.

GARLIC SCAPE AND PISTACHIO PESTO

I small bunch garlic scapes, tops and tough bottoms trimmed

⅓ cup shelled unsalted pistachios

3 tablespoons packed fresh flat-leaf parsley leaves

3 tablespoons packed fresh mint leaves

3 tablespoons packed fresh dill

Zest and juice of 2 lemons

9 small anchovy fillets

½ cup extra-virgin olive oil

Coarse sea salt and freshly ground black pepper

1 Bring a small saucepan of water to a boil. Fill a bowl with ice and water. Cut the garlic scapes into 2-inch lengths. Add to the boiling water and cook until bright green, about 30 seconds. Drain and immediately transfer to the ice water. When cool, drain again. Dry in a salad spinner or by patting with paper towels.

2 In a small skillet, toast the pistachios over high heat, shaking the pan often to prevent the nuts from burning, until golden brown and fragrant, about 3 minutes. Let cool completely.

3 In a food processor or blender, combine the blanched scapes, parsley, mint, dill, lemon zest, lemon juice, anchovies, olive oil, and a pinch of pepper. Puree until smooth, scraping the bowl occasionally. Add the pistachios and pulse until the nuts are very finely chopped. Season with salt.

Ramp greens offer layers of complexity in this super-fast pesto. I serve this with Poached Eggs with Spring Vegetables (page 174), which make good use of the ramp bulbs. It'd also be delicious on eggs simply cooked any way.

MAKES ABOUT
¾ CUP

RAMP AND ALMOND PESTO

4 anchovy fillets

I bunch ramps, greens only

¼ cup raw almonds

¼ teaspoon red pepper flakes

½ cup fresh flat-leaf parsley leaves

½ cup extra-virgin olive oil

Zest and juice of I lemon

2 tablespoons champagne vinegar

Coarse sea salt and freshly ground black pepper

In a food processor, combine the anchovies, ramp greens, almonds, red pepper flakes, and parsley and pulse until finely chopped, scraping the bowl occasionally. Add the olive oil, lemon zest, lemon juice, and vinegar. Process until almost smooth. Season with salt and pepper.

The flavors are Asian, the technique French. That means this is versatile enough for both cuisines. I use it in Steamed Pistou-Rubbed Monkfish Fillets Wrapped in Collards (page 195). It'd also be good with other firm fish or poached chicken. Keep the stems on all the herbs.

MAKES ABOUT
½ CUP

GINGER, MINT, CILANTRO, AND BASIL PISTOU WITH COCONUT OIL

I garlic clove

I tablespoon sliced peeled fresh ginger

I tablespoon sliced jalapeño

½ cup fresh cilantro

½ cup fresh basil

¼ cup fresh flat-leaf parsley

3 tablespoons fresh mint

¼ cup coconut oil, warmed just until liquid

2 tablespoons rice vinegar

½ teaspoon coarse sea salt

Combine all the ingredients in a food processor or blender and puree until smooth, scraping the bowl occasionally. Use immediately.

My twist on the classic Argentinean herb sauce has a bunch of toasted pine nuts thrown in for extra protein, good fats, and terrific nutty flavor. I do a big batch here because it can be kept in the fridge for up to a week. I serve it with Grilled Hanger Steak (page 249) and like to have extra on hand to serve with vegetables or fish.

MAKES ABOUT
2 CUPS

CHIMICHURRI

I bunch cilantro

I bunch basil

I bunch flat-leaf parsley

I garlic clove

I teaspoon red pepper flakes

Zest and juice of I lemon

I tablespoon raw apple cider vinegar

2 cups extra-virgin olive oil

½ cup pine nuts, toasted

Coarse sea salt and freshly ground black pepper

In a blender or food processor, combine the cilantro, basil, parsley, garlic, red pepper flakes, lemon zest, lemon juice, vinegar, and olive oil and pulse until the herbs are coarsely chopped but not pureed. Transfer to a bowl and fold in the pine nuts. Season with salt and pepper.

Coconut oil and jalapeño bring Latin and Asian notes to this cilantro sauce. I serve it with Braised Lamb Shanks in Lettuce Cups (page 240). It'd be great on grilled avocado halves (see page 134) or seared salmon (see page 182), too.

MAKES ABOUT
1½ CUPS

CILANTRO SALSA VERDE

2 cups fresh cilantro, coarsely chopped

I shallot, finely minced

Zest and juice of I lemon

2 tablespoons coconut oil, warmed just until liquid

I tablespoon rice vinegar

I jalapeño, seeded and finely diced

Coarse sea salt and freshly ground black pepper

In a medium bowl, combine the cilantro, shallot, lemon zest, lemon juice, coconut oil, vinegar, and jalapeño. Stir until well mixed, then season with salt and pepper.

Juicy, salty, and a little sour, capers make salsa verde totally satisfying. The sauce was created for Grilled Lamb and Eggplant Kabobs on Rosemary Skewers (page 242), but would be great over fish or pork, too.

MAKES ABOUT 1½ CUPS

MINT AND PARSLEY SALSA VERDE

½ cup fresh mint leaves

½ cup fresh flat-leaf parsley leaves

6 anchovy fillets

2 tablespoons drained capers

2 tablespoons pine nuts

Zest of 1 lemon

¼ garlic clove

½ teaspoon red pepper flakes

1 cup extra-virgin olive oil

Coarse sea salt

In a food processor, combine the mint, parsley, anchovies, capers, pine nuts, lemon zest, garlic, and red pepper flakes and pulse until finely chopped. With the machine running, add the olive oil in a slow, steady stream. Process until smooth. Season with salt.

If you can't find sorrel, use spinach leaves instead and add 3 table-spoons fresh lemon juice to mimic the herb's tartness. This bright sauce cuts through the richness of Perfectly Grilled Lamb Loin Chops (page 229) and would be delicious with seared pork chops (see page 257), too.

MAKES ABOUT
I CUP

SORREL SALSA VERDE

⅔ cup sorrel or spinach leaves

⅓ cup fresh mint leaves

⅓ cup fresh flat-leaf parsley leaves

I tablespoon finely grated lemon zest

I teaspoon red pepper flakes

I garlic clove, thinly sliced

⅓ cup extra-virgin olive oil

Coarse sea salt and freshly ground
black pepper

I tablespoon fresh lemon juice

1 In a blender, combine the sorrel, mint, parsley, lemon zest, red pepper flakes, garlic, and olive oil and puree, scraping down the bowl occasionally, until smooth. Season with salt and pepper.

2 Just before serving, stir in the lemon juice and season with salt and pepper again.

SORREL

Even though this is a leafy green herb, it has a fruity sourness. (Not entirely surprising, since it's related to rhubarb.) The tender leaves in early spring work well raw, and the tougher big leaves that last through summer and fall take on a bitterness best tamed by cooking. Its high potassium level makes it good for circulation, and its high vitamin A and C content boosts your immune system.

Even though I created this for Grilled Avocados (page 134), I also like eating it by the spoonful. Toasted pepitas pop with each bite of the bright grapefruit and herb mix. For a super-light snack, you could wrap it in lettuce cups, too.

MAKES ABOUT 1½ CUPS

GRAPEFRUIT AND JALAPEÑO SALSA

¼ cup pepitas (hulled pumpkin seeds)

1 red grapefruit

½ jalapeño, cut into paper-thin slices on a mandoline

Jacobsen flake finishing sea salt

1 spring garlic or scallion, white part only, very thinly sliced

½ cup fresh cilantro, chopped

1 tablespoon avocado oil

1 In a small skillet, toast the pepitas over high heat, tossing occasionally until golden brown, about 3 minutes. Let cool completely.

2 Trim the top and bottom of the grapefruit, then use a paring knife to cut off all the pith and peel. Holding the grapefruit over a bowl, cut out the segments between the membranes, letting the segments drop into the bowl. Squeeze all the juice you can from the membranes, then discard the membranes.

3 Add the jalapeño and season with salt. Toss well, then fold in the spring garlic, cilantro, avocado oil, and pepitas. Serve immediately.

Whenever cherry tomatoes are in season, I throw together this sauce. Tangy caper berries and the bite of shallots liven up fresh tomatoes and herbs. While the anchovy is optional for vegetarians, I highly recommend it otherwise. It adds a salty complexity. I especially like this sauce on fish, but it's also delicious on vegetables.

MAKES ⅓ CUP

SAUCE VIERGE

¼ cup chopped cherry tomatoes

1 tablespoon chopped caper berries

1 tablespoon minced shallot

½ salted anchovy fillet, minced

1 tablespoon minced fresh flat-leaf parsley

1 tablespoon minced fresh basil

Zest and juice of 1 lemon

¼ cup extra-virgin olive oil

Freshly ground black pepper

Fold all the ingredients together in a small bowl. The sauce can be refrigerated in an airtight container for up to 3 days.

This is my go-to condiment. It's super flavorful and full of good fats. The richness of anchovies and nuts makes it ideal for something with heft, like steak, monkfish, or swordfish. I also spoon it over Perfectly Grilled Halibut (page 188) and toss it with Zucchini Noodles (page 100).

MAKES ABOUT
2 CUPS

CHERRY TOMATO, ANCHOVY, BASIL, AND PISTACHIO SAUCE

I garlic clove, sliced

6 anchovy fillets

¼ cup extra-virgin olive oil

I pint cherry tomatoes, halved

2 tablespoons shelled unsalted pistachios

I tablespoon very thinly sliced red chile

I tablespoon champagne vinegar

2 tablespoons fresh basil leaves, chopped

2 tablespoons fresh tarragon leaves, chopped

Coarse sea salt

1   Put the garlic and anchovies in a mortar and pound with the pestle until everything is well smashed. (If you don't have a mortar and pestle, you can mince everything together while smashing it with the flat side of the knife.)

2   In a large skillet, heat the olive oil over medium-high heat. Add the tomatoes and let sizzle, stirring occasionally, for 1 minute. Add the anchovy mixture and stir well. Add the pistachios and stir well, then add the chile. Add the vinegar, stir well, then remove from the heat.

3   Transfer the mixture to a bowl and stir in the basil and tarragon. Season with salt. Use immediately or refrigerate in an airtight container for up to 2 days. Bring to room temperature before using.

Avocado takes the place of eggs in this aioli, making it super luscious and creamy. I use it in Vietnamese BLT Wraps (page 261) and simply slather it over thick slices of ripe tomato, too.

AVOCADO AIOLI

½ cup avocado oil

½ cup extra-virgin olive oil

I ripe avocado, pitted and peeled

2 garlic cloves

4 cilantro sprigs

I flat-leaf parsley sprig

Zest and juice of 2 lemons

Juice of 2 limes

2 tablespoons white wine vinegar

Coarse sea salt and freshly ground black pepper

1   Combine the avocado oil and olive oil in a liquid measuring cup with a spout.

2   In a food processor or blender, combine the avocado, garlic, cilantro, parsley, lemon zest and juice, lime juice, vinegar, and a generous pinch of salt and pepper and puree until smooth, scraping the bowl occasionally.

3   With the machine running, add the oil blend in a steady stream. Process until emulsified. Season with salt and pepper.

Even though Concord grapes are the base of this sauce, the overall taste ends up savory. That's because I brown the butter until toasty, which also intensifies the ginger's heat. The combination is perfect over Roast Coppa Pork Shoulder (page 258), but would also be fantastic with seared pork chops, steak, or duck breasts. You could also spoon a dollop over yogurt or make it part of a cheese plate, too.

MAKES ABOUT 1½ CUPS

CONCORD GRAPE AND GINGER SAUCE

I pound Concord grapes, removed from stems

I tablespoon grass-fed unsalted butter

I (2-inch) piece fresh ginger (unpeeled), finely chopped

I teaspoon ground cardamom

Coarse sea salt

1 Cut the grapes in half with a sharp paring knife and pick out the seeds with the tip of the knife. Discard the seeds.

2 Put the butter and ginger in a medium skillet and set over medium-low heat. Cook, stirring, until the ginger just turns golden, about 2 minutes.

3 Add the grapes and 2 tablespoons water and stir well. Add the cardamom and stir well. Generously season with salt, stir, and bring to a boil. Reduce the heat to keep the mixture boiling steadily but not furiously. Cook until slightly thickened, about 5 minutes.

4 Remove from the heat and serve warm or at room temperature.

Creamy butter and tart lime juice seal salt and spicy Espelette pepper onto pepitas. After cooking, the pepitas should crisp and dry while they cool. If they're not crunchy when cool, toast them in a 450°F oven until crisp. I sprinkle these all over Celery and Treviso Radicchio Salad (page 45) and just about any other salad. Of course, you can snack on them, too.

MAKES ¼ CUP

SPICED PEPITAS

½ tablespoon grass-fed unsalted butter

¼ cup pepitas (hulled pumpkin seeds)

½ lime

Fine sea salt

Espelette pepper

1   In a small skillet, melt the butter over high heat. Add the pepitas, stirring to coat, and cook, stirring often, until dry, golden brown, and puffed, about 3 minutes. Squeeze the lime over the pepitas, reserving the rind, and stir well for 1 minute. Remove from the heat.

2   Transfer the pepitas to paper towels to drain. Sprinkle immediately with salt and Espelette and zest the lime directly on top. Let cool completely.

Butter and walnuts are really good together because walnuts are bitter and butter is sweet. I add the butter after toasting the walnuts for a minute to keep the sweet cream in it from burning. The salty, crunchy nuts are great over Arugula and Nectarine Salad (page 58) or any other salad, for that matter.

MAKES ½ CUP

BUTTERED SALTED WALNUTS

½ cup walnuts

½ tablespoon grass-fed unsalted butter

Jacobsen flake finishing sea salt

Espelette pepper

1 In a small skillet, cook the walnuts over high heat, tossing occasionally, for 1 minute. Add the butter and cook, tossing and stirring, until the butter melts and the walnuts are well coated, 1 to 2 minutes. Sprinkle with the salt and Espelette.

2 Transfer the nuts to paper towels to drain and cool completely. The nuts will crisp as they cool.

You can make good store-bought ingredients even better. Here, anchovies get covered in fresh oil, along with garlic, thyme, and chile. Not only do you end up with tastier anchovies, but you also have flavorful oil to use for dressing salads or drizzling on roasted vegetables.

MAKES
1 HALF-PINT
JAR

MARINATED ANCHOVIES

1 (2½-ounce) tin anchovies in olive oil

1 garlic clove

3 lemon thyme sprigs

1 dried chile

Extra-virgin olive oil

Transfer the anchovies from the tin to a small jar, leaving the oil behind. Add the garlic, thyme, and chile. Add enough olive oil to cover the solids, then screw on the lid.

Refrigerate for up to 2 months.

When you cook eggs like this, the whites are firmly set and the yolks are just cooked through and still a little creamy. For a firmer yolk, increase the cooking time by 1 minute.

JUST-RIGHT BOILED EGGS

4 large eggs

1 Fill a large bowl with 2 cups ice and 4 cups cold water. Bring 4 cups water to a rolling boil in a medium saucepan.

2 Use a large spoon to carefully add the eggs to the boiling water. Cook for 6½ minutes. As soon as the timer goes off, transfer the eggs to the ice water. Let the eggs cool completely.

3 Carefully peel the eggs and refrigerate in an airtight container for up to 5 days.

My simple trick for infusing quinoa with flavor? Tossing a trio of bay leaf, chile, and thyme into the pot. I make big batches at a time so I always have some on hand to bulk up light, vegetable-centric meals. Use this base for Quinoa Salad with Cucumbers, Herbs, and Tuna with Lemon Honey Mustard Vinaigrette (page 76).

MAKES ABOUT
6 CUPS

AROMATIC TRICOLOR QUINOA

2 cups tricolor quinoa

I bay leaf

I dried chile

2 thyme sprigs

5 cups stock (pages 138 to 143) or water

Coarse sea salt

Rinse the quinoa in a fine-mesh sieve under cold water until the water runs clear. Transfer to a saucepan and add the bay leaf, chile, thyme, stock, and a generous pinch of salt.

Bring to a boil over high heat, then reduce the heat to maintain a low, steady simmer. Cover and cook until cooked through and tender, 20 to 25 minutes. Drain any excess liquid and discard the bay leaf, chile, and thyme.

Use immediately or transfer to an airtight container and refrigerate for up to 5 days.

REAL FOOD HEALS 21-DAY REBOOT

The recipes in this book are perfect for maintaining a healthy diet and are simple to ease into if you're already heading down that path. If you've been eating junk for a long time or most of your life, or even just for the past few weeks, you may want to start with a total reboot. Here's what you've got to do to get on track.

1. No sugar.

- No fruit except blueberries (preferably wild, fresh or frozen), grapefruit, and other tart whole fruit and berries.
- No juice.
- No dried fruit.

2. Keep carbs below 150 grams (5.3 ounces) a day.

- Use a tracker that lets you look at your macros and carb intake.
- Eat healthy carbs from nuts and nonstarchy vegetables, not from grains or starchy vegetables.
- Avoid all legumes.

3. No oxidative oils.

- Avoid all "vegetable" and seed oils like canola, rapeseed, grapeseed, and peanut.
- Use avocado, olive, or coconut oil instead.

4. No processed foods or snacking

- With one big meal in the middle of the day and one good, sensible dinner, your need to snack will be greatly reduced. At first you may feel some hunger as your body craves carbs, but that will subside.

5. Do a high-intensity interval training (HIIT) workout in the morning in a fasted state.

- Start with a 15- to 30-minute warmup of sun salutations and gentle yoga, some jumping jacks, or jump-roping to elevate your heart rate. Then, do one or two Tabata workouts of sprinting, rowing, or cycling. Use a Tabata timer, push full gas for 20 seconds alternating with 10 seconds of recovery.

- Finish with 10 minutes of strength training: plyometrics like push-ups, wall sits, plank, squat hold, or work with heavy weights, and do 3 sets of dead lifts or kettlebell swings.

6. Eat as much *real food* as you want.

- Eat good fats like coconut (oil or fresh flesh or unsweetened desiccated), avocado, grass-fed butter, and pepitas.

- Eat dark leafy vegetables, bitter vegetables, wild fish, pastured meats, whole eggs, and good fats like avocado, grass-fed butter, pepitas, and coconut (oil or fresh flesh or unsweetened desiccated).

7. Eat the following foods in moderation:

- Wild rice, the only acceptable carb on the 21-day reboot

- Sweet potatoes, but only once or twice a week

- Beets, but only once or twice a week and not the same days as sweet potatoes

- Nuts, either raw or dry-roasted with sea salt. The best options are macadamia, almond, walnuts, and hazelnuts, followed by cashews and Brazil nuts. No peanuts! They aren't nuts—they're legumes.

- Stay away from dairy except for ghee (clarified butter) or grass-fed butter. If you are really craving it, only have full-fat dairy.

SAMPLE DAY

On the Real Food Heals 21-Day Reboot, you eat as much *real food* as you want, which may mean you're eating as many as 2,800 calories a day. Counting calories is irrelevant as long as the quality of the calories is high. As your body adapts, you may choose to skip breakfast, but here's a good example of a typical day:

MORNING

- Wake up and drink water.

- If you drink coffee, have it black or with cream or butter. Avoid all espresso drinks unless you are having them black. Avoid almond, soy, oat, hemp, or other nut or seed milks.

- If you're actually hungry, here are two options:

  » Smoothie: Whatever you blend, keep the smoothie pretty savory. It will take time to adjust to this, but you need to keep sugar to a minimum. Try water, ice, apple, kale, avocado, blueberries, coconut oil, almond butter, honey, and ginger.

  » Or Eggs: An example of a good meal would be two fried eggs, bacon, a slice of avocado, and sautéed greens, broccoli, or cabbage.

MIDDAY

- Make a big-ass salad. Try any of the recipes on pages 35 to 95. Or, come up with your own. You want a combination of dark greens; grilled, roasted, or steamed vegetables; seeds; protein; herbs; avocado. If I'm out, I'll modify a salad from a reputable fast-casual joint, asking them to keep out the dairy and grains and adding bacon and avocado for extra fat. I suggest keeping away from dairy initially. Later, if you want, you can add some cheese.

LATE AFTERNOON

- Snack, but only if you must. And if you really have to, here are **three good** options:

  » Nori rolled with avocado, soft-boiled egg, anchovies or good canned tuna, and hot sauce.

  » Almond butter and celery.

  » Small amount of artisanal cured meats or beef jerky.

EVENING

- To maximize weight loss and decrease inflammation, I'd skip alcohol. However, if that's not realistic, have a gin, vodka, or some wine. Stay away from brown liquor and beer, and make sure all mixers are sugar-free and not sodas or juices. (Good luck with that!)

- The best dinner choices are:

  » Sashimi: This is an easy way to eat well on the reboot. Forgo the rice and have vegetable side dishes and miso soup, which is very filling. An alternative to traditional Japanese combinations is salads with raw fish. You'll get plenty of protein and fat without the carbs.

  » Grilled fish, fowl, or meat with vegetables (just not potatoes). Combine the staples on pages 290 to 307 with any of the salads or vegetables.

- For dessert, reward yourself with a few pieces of 75% (or higher) cacao bittersweet dark chocolate.

- The one thing to stay strict about during the reboot is limiting consumption of fruit, alcohol, beets, and sweet potatoes. But the refined carbs (bread, pasta, rice, legumes, and all things crunchy and salty-sweet that come packaged) and refined sugar should be ditched for good. After a while, your body will no longer crave them and you will realize that they make you feel terrible and you won't even want them.

ACKNOWLEDGMENTS

I'm grateful to so many people who've made this book—and the journey to it—a reality and a joy.

Thank you to everyone who helped me create these pages: my co-author Genevieve Ko, agent Kari Stuart, editor Lucia Watson, editorial assistant Nina Caldas, designer Ashley Tucker, production editor Erica Rose, photographer Colin Clark, food stylist Carrie Ann Purcell, food styling assistant Lauren La Penna, prop stylist Martha Bernabe, prop assistants Elvis Meynard, photo shoot social media documenter Jennifer Davidson, publicist Evyn Block, and Avery publicist Anne Kosmoski.

I'm humbled by the praise of those who've written in support of this book. Thank you to Dr. Frank Lipman for your foreword, and to Gwyneth Paltrow, Melissa Hemsley, Jasmine Hemsley, Terry Wahls, Tara Stiles, Daniel Humm, and Marcus Samuelsson.

Thank you to my partners in food, cycling, and philanthropy: Julie Smolyansky and the team from Lifeway Foods; Adele Schober from Breville; Specialized Bicycles; ENVE Composites; The Vanilla Workshop; Ilya and Kasia and the team from Red Beard Bikes; and Adele Nelson, Billy and Debbie Shore, Jenny Dirksen, and the team from Share our Strength.

Thank you to those who helped me transform my body and health and understand how real food heals: Dr. Frank Lipman, Dr. Robin Berzin, Dr. Terry Wahls, Ari Meisel, Jeff Krasno, Schuyler Grant, Jon Gordon, Tim Johnson, Ted King, Andy Levine, and the team from Duvine.

I couldn't have written this book without the support of my restaurants' teams. Every day, I'm thankful for: chef de cuisine Neil Ross, former chef de cuisine Anup Joshi, partner Pamela Stubbs, and general manager and partner Gil Avital.

My colleagues in the industry continue to inspire me. I'm grateful for this community of friends: Amanda Freitag, Marco Canora, George Mendes, Akhtar Nawab, Suzuki-san, April Bloomfield, Andrew Carmellini, Michael Anthony, Bill Telepan, Jeff Mahin, Jason Roberts, Pete Evans, Tom Colicchio, and Jonathan Waxman.

I am always so thankful for the love and support of my family and friends: Tara Mullen and William Lockwood, John Mellquist and Zsuzsa Mitro, Nils Mellquist and Daria Sanford, Marlow Mellquist, William Mellquist, Lynn Juang, Mario Brockman, Louis Somma, William Taylor, Nick Rosen, The Rabbi, Rob Genna Veksler, Whitney Ward, Eli McCoy, Dirk and Jen Shaw, Jim Read, and CJ and Drake the Dog.

Genevieve Ko Acknowledgments

Thank you to Seamus for all the delicious recipes, inspiring knowledge, and generous friendship; to George Mendes for introducing us; to Leslie Stoker and Kari Stuart for cementing our partnership; to Colin, Carrie, and the photography team for stunning images; to Lucia Watson, Nina Caldas, and the whole Avery team for shepherding and championing this book.

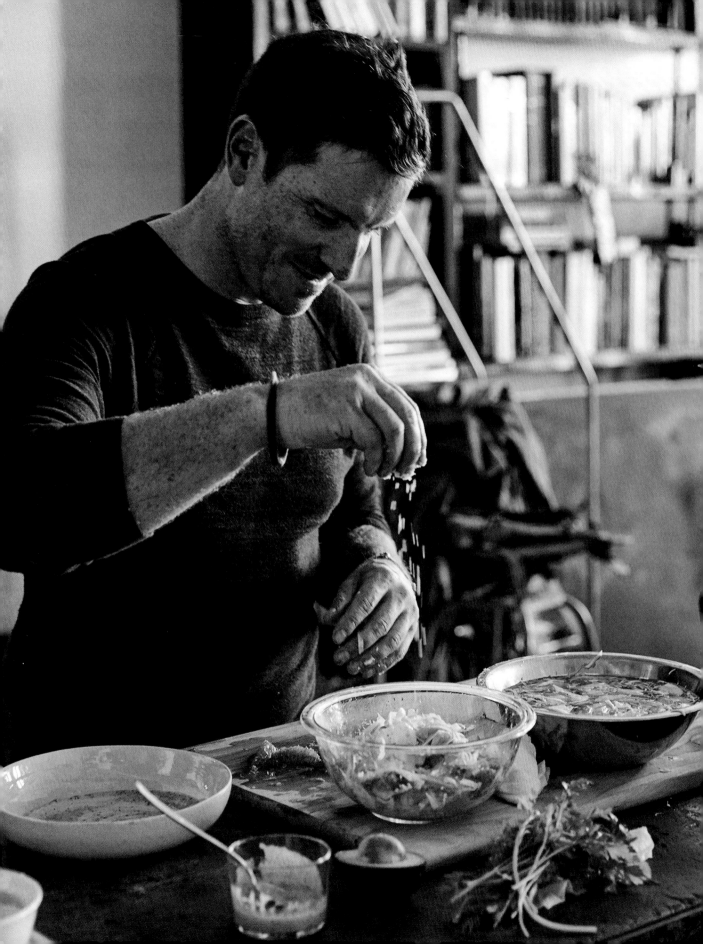

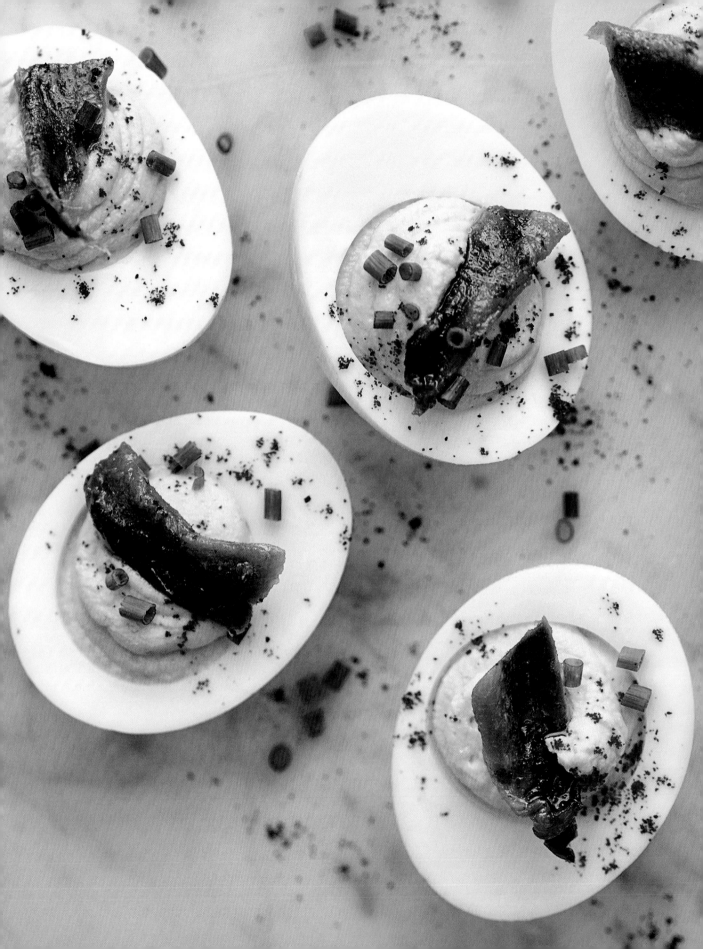

INDEX

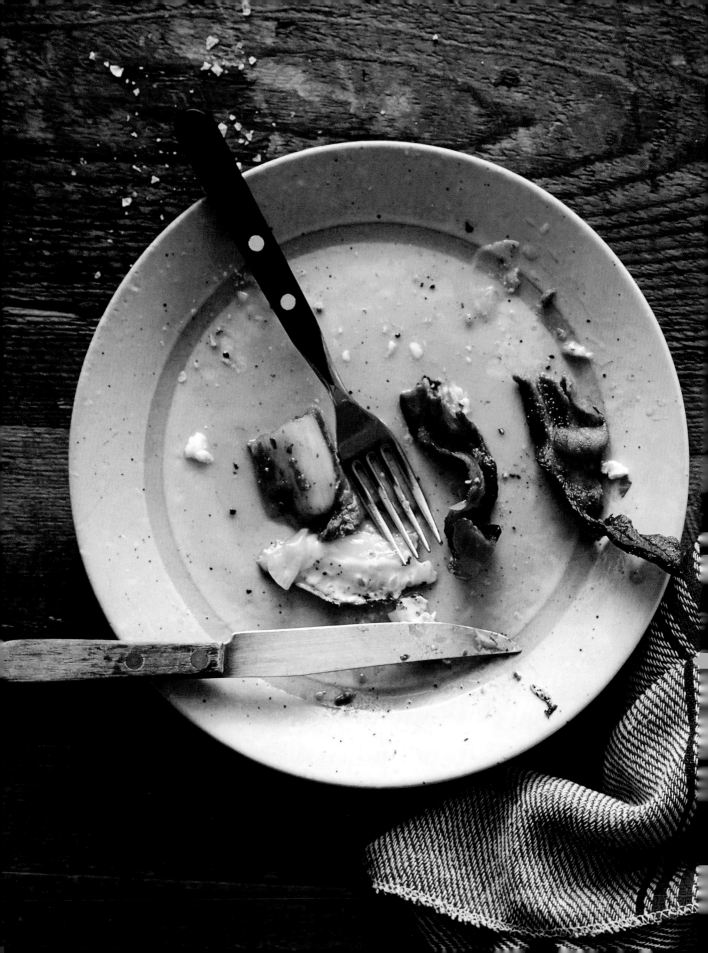